W9-AUI-271

BASIC ESSENTIALS®

Wilderness
First Aid

A FALCON GUIDE®

BASIC ESSENTIALS® SERIES

BASIC ESSENTIALS®
Wilderness First Aid

Third Edition

WILLIAM W. FORGEY, MD

FALCON GUIDE®

GUILFORD, CONNECTICUT
HELENA, MONTANA

AN IMPRINT OF THE GLOBE PEQUOT PRESS

FALCONGUIDE ®

Text and page design by Nancy Freeborn
Illustrations on pages 7, 8, 10, 11, 12, 13, 25, 43, and 63 by Diane Blasius

The Sawyer Accident/Evacuation Record (Appendix A) is reprinted with permission.

Library of Congress Cataloging-in-Publication Data
Forgey, William W., 1942-
  Basic essentials. Wilderness first aid / William W. Forgey. — 3rd ed.
    p. cm.— (Basic essentials)
  ISBN-13: 978-0-7627-4141-0
  ISBN-10: 0-7627-4141-4
  1. Outdoor medical emergencies. 2. First aid in illness and injury. I. Title.
  RC88.9.O95F673 2006
  616.02′52—dc22   2006048697

Manufactured in the United States of America
Third Edition/First Printing

To Kurt Avery of Clearwater, Florida, the CEO of Sawyer Products and a great soccer dad. His work in promoting and developing new technologies in insect repellents, sunblocks, and snakebite care has benefited all who venture outdoors.

Contents

Injury Reference Chart

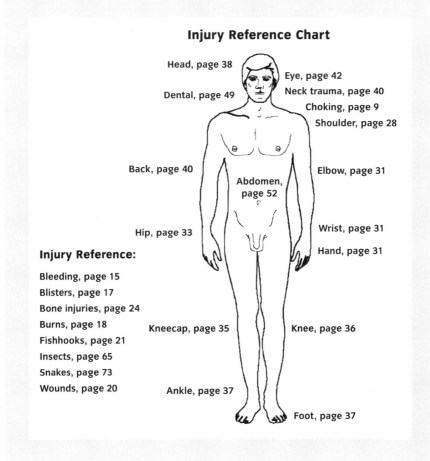

Head, page 38

Eye, page 42

Dental, page 49

Neck trauma, page 40

Choking, page 9

Shoulder, page 28

Back, page 40

Abdomen, page 52

Elbow, page 31

Hip, page 33

Wrist, page 31

Hand, page 31

Injury Reference:

Bleeding, page 15

Blisters, page 17

Bone injuries, page 24

Burns, page 18

Fishhooks, page 21

Insects, page 65

Snakes, page 73

Wounds, page 20

Kneecap, page 35

Knee, page 36

Ankle, page 37

Foot, page 37

Illness Reference Chart

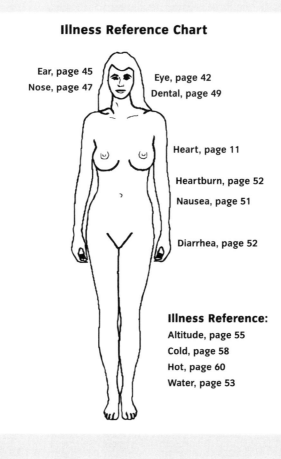

Ear, page 45

Nose, page 47

Eye, page 42

Dental, page 49

Heart, page 11

Heartburn, page 52

Nausea, page 51

Diarrhea, page 52

Illness Reference:

Altitude, page 55

Cold, page 58

Hot, page 60

Water, page 53

Introduction

Virtually every method of handling injury and illness in the wilderness is different from what you would expect in an urban environment. The remoteness from "civilization," the lack of readily available medical assistance, and the difficulty of having to handle serious injuries on your own—often for many hours—can be daunting if you are not prepared. Thus, a book on first aid in the wilderness is much more than a standard first-aid text. It can help ready you to meet the challenges of stabilizing injuries in remote wilderness areas.

While standard first-aid classes can provide a good basic introduction to helping injured individuals, the special techniques described in this book are taught in wilderness first-aid classes. You can learn more about these classes by checking the Wilderness Medical Society Web page at www.wms.org, at this book's supporting Web page at http://adventure-media.com, or by visiting www.docforgey.com or www.docforgeytravelmedicine.com. If you haven't already taken a CPR course, it is also a good idea to do so. Classes can be obtained through your local American Red Cross chapter.

TERMS USED IN THIS BOOK

Throughout this book I have used the terms "evacuate," "treatment," and "return." This terminology is used in wilderness medicine. Understanding what these terms mean in relationship to treating an injured individual is crucial.

Evacuation is an important topic in wilderness first aid. It means to take or have a person taken to a facility where professional medical care can be administered. Most often this is an emergency room in an emergency department at a hospital. There are two types of evacuation: self-evacuation and assisted evacuation. In self-evacuation the party with the victim takes care of the entire procedure. This includes caring and feeding for the victim as well as helping move or carry the individual if need be. In an assisted evacuation, sometimes called an "outside" evacuation or "rescue," help is requested from outside sources, such a country sheriff or search-and-rescue teams. These people will aid in the evacuation or entirely take over the responsibility of care and movement of the individual.

It is important to know when to evacuate. This procedure is often very expensive, time consuming, and obviously disrupts or ends a trip into the wilderness. Throughout this book I have indicated when an evacuation of a patient is warranted. Always try to self-evacuate if possible. Self-evacuation shortens the length of time it takes to reach professional medical care. It is also socially responsible to attempt to take care of your own party and not to rely on rescue by others, unless it is apparent that the procedure is beyond your capability to handle safely.

At times evacuation is not indicated. Many conditions can be safely treated by the party. Treatment might be aimed at a temporary fix of a problem—something that will help the victim be safe and comfortable so that she can finish the trip and then seek professional care once she is home. An example would be the treatment of a small second-degree burn. At other times, the treatment will be definitive and no further care will be needed after returning home. An example of this would be a decongestant for a stuffy nose that responds well and clears.

BE PREPARED

It would seem that a trip into remote areas would mandate carrying a first-aid kit that could solve all of the possible horrible things that could happen. The great wilderness writers such as Cliff Jacobson have always emphasized that the most important piece of equipment for wilderness travel is not "things" but the "information between one's ears." There is no aspect of wilderness travel that concurs with this attitude more than wilderness first aid.

While it is possible to improvise to a great extent, an appropriate first-aid kit is one of the essentials that should be brought on any wilderness outing. The kit that will be the most compact will be the one that uses both multifunctional and cross-functional components. This means that each item will be used for more than one particular purpose and that various components can be substituted for the same purpose.

To choose the items for your first-aid kit, you should try to anticipate the most likely serious events that could occur and carry only items that you know how to use. Consider the weight, cost, bulk, and availability of components. You should also take into consideration the number in the party, length of trip, degree of risk anticipated, and whether or not people beyond those of the immediate party will be treated.

The following kits contain the type of supplies you should bring with you on your trip. All of the items listed can be obtained without prescriptions at drugstores.

Basic Backpacking Kit

This kit is ideal for one person going backpacking. It is about as light as kits get, yet will handle most problems that a single hiker might encounter. Pack this kit in a small, sealable plastic bag.

- 3 gel dressings (such as Spenco 2nd Skin with adhesive dressing or gel-padded Curad or J&J dressings)
- 4 ibuprofen 200 mg tablets for pain, inflammation, fever
- 4 decongestant-antihistamine tablets (such as Tavist-D, Actifed, or equivalent)

Basic Wilderness First-Aid Kit

This basic kit should be adequate to care for four to six people on a two-week wilderness trip. Experience will demonstrate that many of the bandages will be used in the early part of the trip, while the medications tend to be required later. On subsequent trips adjust quantities of these items to match your experience. Pack this kit in a brightly colored, water-resistant stuff sack for both protection of contents and to make finding it easier in an emergency.

- 5 2"x 2" Spyroflex Blister Dressings (These versatile bandages can be used to replace Band-Aids, stitches, and coverings. They cause blood to clot, provide water-resistant protection, and act as a barrier against outside contamination, making these bandages the most versatile available. They can be kept in place for up to seven days.)
- 1 Sam Splint—malleable aluminum/foam splint
- 1 3" elastic bandage for sprains, contusions, and holding splints and bandages in place
- 1 4" elastic bandage
- 1 pair protective gloves
- 1 disposable CPR mask
- 6 povidone-iodine antiseptic swabs or ½ oz. Hibiclens surgical scrub
- 4 3"x 3" sterile gauze pads
- 4 Q-tips
- 1 pair tweezers
- 1 ½ oz. tube dibucaine 1% ointment for anesthesia, itch

- 1 ½ oz. tube triple-antibiotic ointment
- 1 ½ oz. tube antifungal cream
- 6 laxative tablets for constipation
- 6 loperamide 2 mg tablets for diarrhea
- 6 meclizine 25 mg tablets for nausea, motion sickness
- 8 ibuprofen 200 mg tablets for pain, inflammation, fever
- 8 decongestant-antihistamine tablets (such as Tavist-D, Actifed, or equivalent)
- 8 Benadryl (diphenhydramine) 25 mg capsules for antihistamine, cough suppression, muscle spasm, allergy reactions
- 1 Sawyer Extractor

Now that you have a kit all packed, learn the skills to use it and the wilderness travel techniques so well that you can perform first aid in the wilderness.

FOR MORE INFORMATION

A further discussion of the techniques of handling wilderness related injuries and illness—particularly prolonged care when evacuation or rescue may not be an option—can be found in my book *Wilderness Medicine*, fifth edition. Another excellent book on the assessment and transport of the patient for evacuation is *Medicine for the Backcountry* by Buck Tilton and Frank Hubble. For cold-weather-related injuries, refer to my book *Basic Essentials Hypothermia* (The Globe Pequot Press). See appendix B for details.

CHAPTER ONE

Initial Survey

Your worst fears are realized: An accident has happened. And what makes it even more alarming, it has occurred in a remote wilderness area, far from help. Regardless of the severity of the accident, if you follow a series of well-established steps, you will have done what is necessary to preserve life, to minimize pain or further injury, and to help prepare the victim for evacuation. The first-aid steps that you may be familiar with that and are correct for an urban environment will have to be modified to handle an injury that has occurred in a remote location.

SECURE THE SCENE

On reaching an accident victim, the first duty in an urban environment is to activate the emergency medical services by calling 911. Afterward the initial care consists of an urgent, simultaneous attempt to examine the patient and correct life-threatening injuries relating to breathing, heartbeat, and blood loss, while at the same time protecting the victim from a possible spine injury.

In the wilderness, however, before assessing the patient, you must assess the scene! Make sure that it is safe and that falling rock, floods, or other dangers will not hurt you or others. If the area is dangerous, you will have to immediately remove the patient to a safer location and keep other persons away from the scene to prevent them from getting hurt. Accidents tend to multiply! Some dangers are difficult to see or might be delayed in onset. For example, while treating a sprained knee, don't fail to notice if other members of your party are becoming cold from inactivity and thus at risk for hypothermia.

AIRWAY

After evaluating the scene, the next step is to find out whether or not the victim is having difficulty breathing.

Check the airway: If the victim can talk, his airway is functioning. In an unconscious patient, place your ear next to his nose/mouth and your hand on his chest and look, listen, and feel for air movement.

No air movement: Check to see if the tongue is blocking the airway by pushing down on the forehead while lifting the chin. In case of possible neck injury, the airway can be opened without movement of the neck by lifting the jaw.

Still no air movement: Pinch his nose and seal your mouth over his; try to force air into his lungs. Very lightweight, disposable cardiopulmonary resuscitation (CPR) masks are available that provide sanitary protection.

Still no air movement: Perform the Heimlich maneuver (see page 9). Once you are able to establish air movement, continue CPR until the victim can breathe on his own.

CIRCULATION

Check circulation by placing several of your fingertips lightly into the hollow below the angle of the patient's jaw to feel for a pulse.

No pulse: Start CPR (see page 12).

SEVERE BLEEDING

Check quickly for severe blood loss. Check visually and with your hands. Slide your hand under the victim to ensure that blood is not leaking into the ground and check inside bulky garments for hidden blood loss.

Severe bleeding: Use direct pressure (see page 15).

NECK

During the initial survey keep the patient's head and neck as still as possible if you suspect a neck injury. Your suspicions should be high if the patient is unconscious or had an accident, such as a fall or significant blow to the head. See treatment of cervical spine injuries, pages 40–41.

CHAPTER TWO

Focused Survey

While the purpose of the initial survey is to hastily find and correct life-threatening conditions, the focused survey is an attempt to identify all of the medical problems that the patient might have. This requires a thorough examination, because sometimes an obvious injury can be distracting. A broken bone may prevent both you and the victim from noticing a less painful but potentially more serious injury elsewhere.

The only way to perform a focused survey is to do it thoroughly, using both your vision and sense of touch, asking simple questions, and being methodical in the approach. Sense of touch is important. While sliding your hand under the vic-

TABLE 1

General techniques of a Focused Survey

1. Start at the head and work your way down the victim's body.

2. Move the patient as little as possible and try not to aggravate known injuries while looking for others.

3. Constantly communicate with the patient during the examination, even if she seems unconscious.

4. Look for damage, even cutting away clothing if necessary to visualize suspected injuries.

5. Ask about pain, discomfort, and abnormal sensations constantly during the exam.

6. Gently feel all relevant body parts for abnormalities.

tim, you might find areas of tenderness or considerable blood loss that would otherwise go unnoticed. It is surprising how much blood can be absorbed into snow or sand under a wounded victim and not be noticed until your hand encounters it.

The mission of the focused survey is not only to discover medical problems but also to record and keep track of them during periodic reassessments. The most significant difference between wilderness first aid and standard urban first aid is that the focused survey must also lead to treatment protocols.

This methodical examination should generally start at the head and work its way to the feet. With children, however, you might want to start with the legs. (Children are sometimes frightened by movement toward their heads.) Generally, starting at the head is best.

VITAL SIGNS

While even accurate measurements of the body's functions will not indicate what is wrong with a patient, the second and subsequent measurements indicate how the patient is progressing. The severity of the accident will determine how often you should take the vital signs, but certainly close monitoring of the patient should be continued until she is "out of the woods."

Vital signs consist of several elements:

Level of Consciousness

Is the patient alert, does she respond only to verbal or painful stimulus, or is she unresponsive?

Pulse

Check and record rate, rhythm, and quality (thready, normal, or bounding) of pulse.

Respirations

Note the rate, rhythm, and quality (labored, with pain, flaring of nostrils, or noise such as snores, squeaks, gurgles, or gasps).

Skin

Check its color and note whether it is hot or cold and moist or dry.

Blood Pressure

This can be taken with a stethoscope and blood pressure cuff or by estimating.

If you can feel a pulse in the radial artery at the wrist, the top (systolic) pressure is probably at least 80 mm Hg. If you can only feel the femoral pulse in the groin, the pressure is no lower than 70 mm Hg. When only the carotid pulse in the neck is palpable, the systolic is probably at least 60 mm Hg. Normal systolic blood pressures range from 100 to 140. Low systolic blood pressures with normal pulses (say the 70 to 85 beats per minute range) are safe. But an increased pulse rate with a low pressure is an indication of shock.

MEDICAL HISTORY

Ask about the patient's allergies, the medications that she is taking, her medical history, her last food or drink, and about the events that led up to the accident. If she is in pain ask: What provokes it? Does it radiate? How severe is it? What type is it (burning, sharp, dull)? What time did it start?

PHYSICAL EXAMINATION

Head

Look for damage, discoloration, and blood or fluid draining from ears, nose, and mouth. Ask about loss of consciousness, pain, or any abnormal sensations. Feel for lumps or other deformities.

Loss of consciousness, see page 4.
Ear trauma, see page 45.
Eye trauma, see page 42.
Nose trauma, see page 47.
Mouth trauma, see page 49.

Neck

Look for obvious damage or deviation of the windpipe (trachea). Ask about pain and discomfort. Feel along the cervical spine for a pain response.

Cervical spine trauma, see page 40.
Breathing difficulty, see page 9.

Chest

Compress the ribs from both sides, as if squeezing a birdcage, keeping your hands wide to prevent the possibility of too much direct pressure on fractures. Look for damage or deformities. Ask about pain. Feel for instability. (Instability can be detected by an unusual movement of the rib cage when it is pressed upon.)

Abdomen

With hands spread wide, press gently on the abdomen. Look for damage. Ask about pain and discomfort. Feel for rigidity, distention, or muscle spasms.

Abdominal pain, see page 51.

Back

Slide your hands under the patient, palpating as much of the spine as possible.

Spine trauma, see page 40.

Pelvis/Hip

Place your hands on the top front of the pelvis on both sides (the iliac crests), pressing gently down, and pulling toward the midline of the body. Ask about pain. Feel for instability.

Hip or pelvis pain, see page 33.

Legs

Surround each leg with both hands and run your hands from the groin down to the toes, squeezing as you go. Note especially if there is a lack of circulation, sensation, or motion in the toes.

Bone injury, see fractures on pages 26–27, 34–37.

Shoulders and Arms

With hands wide, squeeze each shoulder and run your hands down the arms to the fingers. Check for circulation, sensation, and motion in the fingers.

Shoulder trauma, see page 28.

CHAPTER THREE

Shock

Shock is a deficiency in oxygen reaching the brain and other tissues as a result of decreased circulation. If possible, identify and treat the underlying cause of the shock. The initial and focused surveys and history may well elicit the cause of shock, and appropriate treatment can be devised from the methods listed in this book.

Shock can be caused by burns, electrocution, hypothermia, bites, stings, bleeding, fractures, pain, hypothermia, high-altitude cerebral edema, illness, rough handling, allergic reaction (anaphylaxis), head injury, loss of adequate heart strength, or dehydration from sweating, vomiting, or diarrhea. Each of these underlying causes is discussed separately in this text.

Shock can progress through several stages before resulting in death. The first phase is called the "compensatory stage," during which the body attempts to counter the damage by increasing its activity level. Arteries constrict and the pulse rate increases, thus maintaining the blood pressure. The next phase is called the "progressive stage," when suddenly the blood pres-

Figure 1
Position of fingers to check for the carotid artery pulse

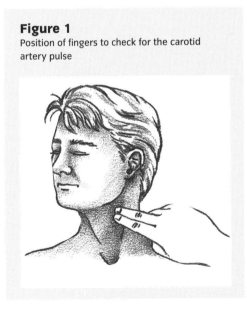

sure drops and the patient becomes worse, often swiftly. When the patient has reached the "irreversible stage," vital organs have suffered so profoundly from loss of oxygen that death occurs even with aggressive treatment.

Consider the possibility of shock in any victim of an accident or when significant illness develops. Ensure that an adequate airway is established (see further discussion under rescue breathing, page 12). Make sure the heart is beating. Place your hand over the carotid artery (figure 1) to obtain the pulse. In compensatory shock the patient will have a weak, rapid pulse. In adults the pulse rate will be over 140, in children 180 beats per minute. If there is doubt about a pulse being present, listen to the bare chest. If there isn't a heartbeat present, begin CPR (see page 12). Elevate the legs to 45 degrees to obtain a better return of blood to the heart and head (figure 2). However, if there has been a severe head injury, keep the person flat. If he has trouble breathing, elevate the chest and head to a comfortable position. Protect the patient from the environment with insulation underneath and shelter up above. Strive to make him comfortable. Watch your spoken and body language. Reassure without patronizing, and let nothing that you say or do cause the injured person increased distress.

Shock due to severe allergic reactions is called "anaphylactic shock" and is discussed on page 66.

Figure 2
Shock treatment position

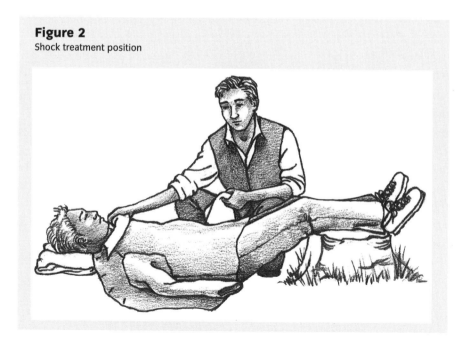

CHAPTER FOUR

Difficulty Breathing

It has been stated that you can live three minutes without air, three days without water, three weeks without food, and three months without love. Some feel that their limit might be stretched to four, while others feel shorter periods might be lethal. Without question, adequate respiration is the most significant demand of a living creature. When respiratory difficulties start, it's urgent to find the reason and alleviate it. When they stop, reestablishing the airflow is critical.

FOREIGN BODY AIRWAY OBSTRUCTION

If a conscious adult seems to be having distressed breathing, ask "Are you choking?" If she apparently is, perform an abdominal thrust or the Heimlich maneuver to relieve foreign-body airway obstruction or choking. If the victim is standing or sitting, stand behind and wrap your arms around the patient (figure 3), proceeding as follows: Make a fist with one hand. Place the thumb side of the fist against the victim's abdomen, in the midline slightly above the navel and well below the breastbone. Grasp your fist with the other hand. Press the fist into the victim's abdomen with a quick, upward thrust. Each new thrust should be a separate and distinct movement. It may be necessary to repeat the thrust multiple times to clear the airway. If the person is obese or pregnant, use chest thrusts in the same manner as just described, but with the hands around the lower chest.

If the victim becomes unconscious and is on the ground, the victim should be placed on her back, face up. In civilization activate the EMS system. Perform a tongue-jaw lift, followed by a finger sweep to remove the object. Open the airway and try to ventilate. If still obstructed, reposition the head and try to ventilate again. Give up to five abdominal thrusts, then repeat the tongue-jaw lift, finger sweep, and attempt ventilation. Repeat these steps until effective.

To perform an abdominal thrust with the patient on the ground, the rescuer kneels astride the victim's thighs. The rescuer places the heel of one hand against the victim's abdomen, in the midline slightly above the navel and well below the breastbone, and the second hand directly on top of the first. The rescuer then presses into the abdomen with quick upward thrusts.

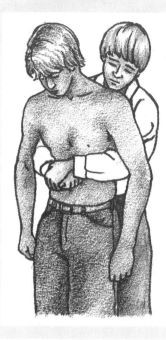

Figure 3
The Heimlich maneuver

CHAPTER FIVE

Heart Attack

Chest heaviness or pain with exertion; pain or ache radiating into the neck or arms; sweating, clammy, pale appearance; shortness of breath—are all classic symptoms of a person having an inadequate oxygen supply to the heart. The pain is called angina, and the event is known as an acute coronary syndrome or heart attack.

Figure 4
A heart attack victim usually can breathe better sitting up.

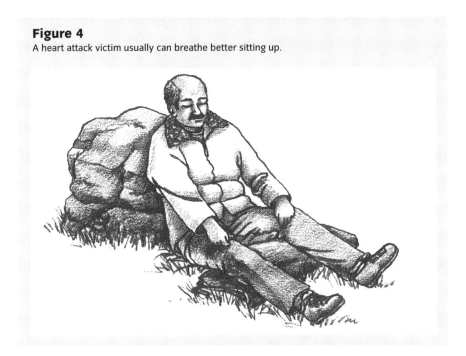

Place the patient in a semisitting position (figure 4). If shock develops, position the patient's head down and feet up to prevent a further drop in blood pressure and further decrease in blood supply to the heart. If the group has any aspirin, give the person 324 mg (a normal-size tablet). If available give the person a nitroglycerine 0.4 mg tablet under the tongue every ten minutes as long as the blood pressure is above 100 mm Hg. If you can feel the person's pulse in the thumb side of the wrist, the pressure should be at or above that level. If the group has any clopidogrel (Plavix), give the person four of the 75 mg tablets immediately. If the group has any metaprolol (Tenormin) or atenolol (Toprol), give 25 mg every six hours beginning six hours after the onset of pain, unless the heart rate is below 60 beats per minute or the blood pressure is below 100. The above are new reperfusion techniques as taught in the *Wilderness Medical Society Practice Guidelines for Wilderness Emergency Care* (Globe Pequot, 2006); these techniques can be lifesaving in a wilderness area. Call as soon as possible for evacuation to medical care.

Tell the person to cough deeply and repetitively if the patient feels he is about to faint. If the person becomes unresponsive, give a thump on the chest. If still unresponsive, start CPR.

ADULT ONE-RESCUER CPR/RESCUE BREATHING

If the person is not breathing normally, begin by opening the airways. The head-tilt, chin-lift method is the proper technique for opening the airway in an unconscious person (figure 5). Pinch the victim's nose and cover his mouth with yours. Blow until you see his chest rise. Give two breaths with each lasting one second.

Figure 5
Opening the airway

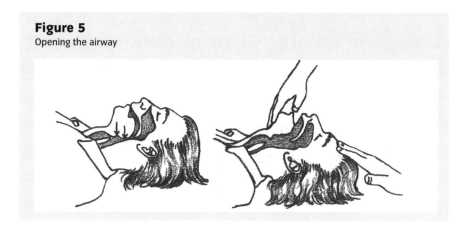

If the victim does not start breathing, coughing, or moving after the two breaths, start chest compressions. Push down on the chest 1½ to 2 inches thirty times at the rate of one hundred compressions per minute. Push down right between the nipples. Figure 6 shows the position of the hands and rescuer when performing chest compressions during CPR.

Continue with two breaths and thirty pumps until help arrives. In the wilderness if the patient does not respond to thirty minutes of CPR, and there is no possibility of professional rescue help arriving, it is appropriate to quit further treatment.

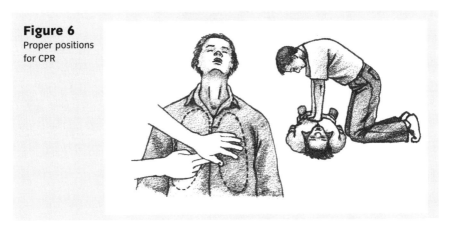

Figure 6
Proper positions for CPR

Learning CPR is an important skill that every person should master. The only way to learn this technique is to take a CPR course—it cannot be properly self-taught.

CHAPTER SIX

Fever/Pain/Itch

These symptoms always indicate that something is wrong. They may go away without treatment, but if fever or significant pain continues longer than twenty-four hours, it is reasonable to stop the trip and return to civilization. In addition to the medications recommended on pages xv and xvi of the introduction, a cold cloth can be applied to treat all three of these problems by providing some relief.

CHAPTER SEVEN

Wilderness Wound Care

Part of the initial survey is to identify and stop life-threatening bleeding. In remote areas care will also include cleaning the wound and protecting it, promoting healing, reducing pain, and minimizing any decrease in function.

Evacuate: In general it is not necessary to evacuate a wound victim, as generally the problem can be adequately handled as indicated above. However, there are times when evacuation or at least termination of a trip is indicated.

An urgent evacuation is advisable for: 1) severe animal bites or bites from potentially rabid animals; 2) deep or highly contaminated wounds with a high risk of infection (any wound contaminated by water that comes from agricultural runoff is highly contaminated); 3) wounds that open to fractures or to joint spaces; 4) infected wounds; and 5) wounds associated with severe blood loss.

Return: Terminate the trip for wounds that, while not urgent, severely limit an individual's ability to participate and require closure for cosmetic reasons (such as wounds on the face). Delayed primary closure of facial wounds can be performed in three to five days if the wound is kept clean with daily packing.

CUTS/BLEEDING

Direct pressure is the best way to stop bleeding—in fact pressure alone can stop bleeding from amputated limbs! Your medical kit should have a pair of barrier (protective) gloves to help prevent contact with blood and the possible germs it might carry (such as hepatitis B and AIDS). When the accident first occurs, immediately use direct pressure to stop the bleeding. If you do not have gloves, try to protect yourself by using cloth, plastic food bags, or anything else available to separate yourself from direct blood contact. Direct pressure may have to be applied for five, ten, even thirty minutes. Apply it as long as it takes! With the blood stopped, and the victim on the ground in the shock-treatment position, the actual emergency is over. Her life is safe for now, and you have bought time to gather together various items that you need to care for the wound.

In the first-aid management of a wound, the next step is simply bandaging and then transporting the victim to professional medical care. Further care in a remote area depends upon the length of time that it will take to get to a doctor. Simply binding the wound in a clean bandage—or in the case of an open, gaping wound, covering it with a wet-to-dry dressing—is appropriate if the time to professional care is two days or less.

A wet-to-dry dressing is made by wetting a sterile gauze pad from your medical kit with sterile, or at least drinkable, water (see page 53) and applying it directly to the wound. This means that you will be packing the inside of a large wound with a damp bandage. A dry overdressing is applied as a cover and taped or held secure with an elastic bandage. This dressing should be changed every twenty-four hours.

If it will be longer than two days to definitive medical care, then further care of the wound becomes essential. It must be thoroughly cleaned; any impaled objects need to be removed, and wound closure may be attempted.

Cleaning Cuts

Adequate cleansing of cuts (lacerations) requires flushing with clean water. Ideally the water should be applied with great force, thus dislodging any blood clots, debris, and associated germ contamination. An irrigating syringe is ideal for this purpose. Without it you will have to do the best that you can, perhaps by placing the water in a clean plastic bag, puncturing a small hole in it, and squeezing the bag forcefully to jet water out into the wound. Using sterile gauze from your kit to scrub the wound while irrigating is also a helpful but painful cleansing technique.

Surgical scrub solutions, such as Betadine (1 percent povidone iodine) or Hibiclens (0.5 percent chlorhexidine gluconate), are also helpful in cleaning a wound, but they must be thoroughly rinsed out of the wound. A *very* mild soap solution can be made using your dish or hand soap, but make it on the mild side rather than too strong, and also be sure to irrigate it all out of the wound.

Wound cleaning is a painful process, but sometimes it can be made less painful if done immediately after the wound has occurred (this is seldom possible) or if an ice pack or chemical cold pack is temporarily applied prior to cleaning (also seldom possible and not all that much help). Work quickly—but thoroughly—to minimize pain. Once the cleaning is completed, bleeding must again be stopped by direct pressure and the wound must be covered with sterile dressing.

Wounds that are still contaminated—as well as high-risk wounds such as animal bites and puncture wounds—should be packed with a wet-to-dry dressing. If the wound apparently has been well cleaned, and particularly if it will take longer than two days to reach professional care, closure with strips of tape can be attempted. Any technique that holds the wound edges together will be adequate. Sometimes simply splinting or wrapping the area will result in closure. Do not tape the edges too tightly, or this will cause puckering of the wound. A small gap in the edges of the wound is acceptable, as the skin can grow across, but puckers or inverted skin edges fail to heal well.

FRICTION BLISTERS

Two of the most common outdoor injuries are friction blisters and minor thermal burns. These injuries always occur early in a trip. New equipment will rub, and novice campers often burn themselves when cooking over a campfire.

An easily obtainable substance has revolutionized the prevention and care of friction blisters. The material is Spenco 2nd Skin, generally available in the footwear section of camping stores. Made from an inert, breathable gel consisting of 4 percent polyethylene oxide and 96 percent water, it feels cold and wet when applied to your skin. The blister kit and padding kit contain adhesive knit tape needed to fasten the 2nd Skin gel to your skin. The tape and gel come in various sizes. The package is watertight but labeled nonsterile. The gel has three valuable properties that make it so useful: It will remove all friction between two moving surfaces (hence its use in prevention); it cleans and deodorizes wounds by absorbing blood, serum, or pus; and its cooling effect is very soothing, which aids in pain relief.

After opening the sealed package, you will find the Spenco 2nd Skin sandwiched between two sheets of cellophane. Remove the cellophane from the side to be applied to the wound or hot spot (the stage before a friction blister develops). It must be secured to the wound with the adhesive knit bandage.

If a friction blister has developed, it will have to be lanced. Cleanse with soap or surgical scrub and open along an edge with a sharp knife blade. After forcing out the fluid, apply a fully stripped piece of 2nd Skin. Remove the cellophane from one side, then apply it to the wound. Once the piece is on the skin surface, remove the cellophane from the outside edge. Over this you will need to place the adhesive knit. The bandage must be kept moist with clean water. Change the dressing daily. The contents of this package *are* actually sterile, but the manufacturer does not indicate a shelf life, so sterility cannot be guaranteed. This product is a valuable addition to your medical kit.

THERMAL BURNS

As soon as possible, remove the source of the burn. Quickly immerse the burned area into cool water, if possible, as this will help eliminate additional heat that may be generated by scalding water, burning fuels, or clothing. Or suffocate the flames with anything available, such as clothing or even sand.

Treatment of burns depends upon the extent (percent of the body covered) and the depth (degree) of the injury. The percent of the body covered is estimated by referring to the "rule of nines," as indicated in figure 7. For example: An entire arm equals 9 percent of the body surface area, therefore the burn of just one side of the forearm would equal about 2 percent. The proportions are slightly different for children.

Severity of burns is indicated by degree. *First degree* (superficial) will have redness and be dry and painful. *Second degree* (partial skin thickness) will be moist and painful and have blister formation with reddened bases. *Third degree* (deep) involves the full thickness of the skin and extends into the subcutaneous tissue with charring, loss of substance, or discoloration. These severe burns are frequently not painful due to nerve destruction, although there will be painful lesions of second- and first-degree burns surrounding the area.

The field treatment of burns has also been revolutionized by the development of Spenco 2nd Skin. It is the perfect substance to use on first-, second-, or third-degree burns. Its cooling effect relieves pain, while its sterile covering absorbs fluid easily from the wound. If applied to a charred third-degree burn, it provides a sterile cover that does not have to be changed. When the patient arrives at a hospital, it can easily be removed in a whirlpool bath.

Figure 7
The rule of nines picture for determining the percentage of a body covered by burns

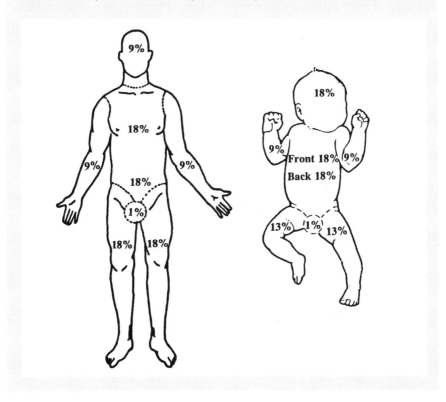

Return: Burn patients can generally be managed quite well if the burn is not worse than second degree and as long as it does not cover more than 15 percent of the body surface area of an adult (10 percent of a child). **Evacuate:** If burns are more extensive than that, or if they involve the face or include more than one joint of the hand, obtain professional treatment. The management will be as above, but in addition, treat the patient for shock during the evacuation (see page 7).

ABRASIONS

An abrasion is the loss of surface skin due to a scraping injury. The best treatment is cleansing with surgical scrub or mild soap and an application of triple-antibiotic ointment (available over the counter at your local pharmacy).

The Spenco 2nd Skin with adhesive knit bandage mentioned on page 17 makes an excellent dressing for abrasions. This type of wound oozes profusely, but the 2nd Skin bandaging allows rapid healing, excellent protection, and considerable pain relief. Avoid the use of rubbing alcohol as it tends to damage the tissue and cause excessive pain. Lacking first-aid supplies, cleanse gently with mild detergent and protect from dirt, bugs, and so forth, the best you can.

BRUISES

Large bruises are a result of a contusion or blunt injury. Treat contusions during the first forty-eight hours with cold compresses or cold-water immersion and a compression dressing—to limit bleeding and to provide pain relief. Apply cold for one-half hour every two hours, but obviously avoid cold injury. After seventy-two hours, apply warm, moist cloths to increase the circulation and aid in healing.

Large bruised areas, especially when swollen, may indicate a large amount of blood loss or a significant underlying injury. Treat people with such injuries for possible shock (see page 7).

Do not drain large, swollen bruise areas. This serves no purpose and can cause bleeding and infection.

Pain or swelling near a bone may mean that a broken bone has occurred (see pages 26–27).

PUNCTURE WOUNDS

Allow puncture wounds to bleed briefly, thus encouraging an automatic release of bacteria from the wound. If available, apply suction with the Sawyer Extractor (venom suction device illustrated in figure 8) immediately and continue the vacuum for two to three minutes. However, if bleeding is brisk, immediately apply direct pressure (see page 15). Cleanse the wound area with surgical scrub or soapy water and apply triple-antibiotic ointment to the surrounding skin surface. Do not tape

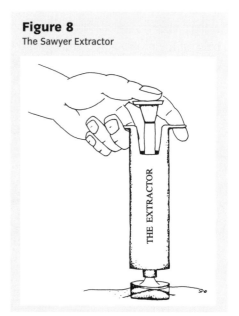

Figure 8
The Sawyer Extractor

THE EXTRACTOR

the wound shut, but start warm compress applications for twenty minutes every two hours for the next two days. These soaks should be as warm as the patient can tolerate without danger of burning the skin. Large pieces of cloth work best, such as undershirts, as they hold the heat longer. Cover with a clean cloth. If sterile items are in short supply, they need not be used on this type of wound. Use clean clothes or boil such items and allow to cool and dry before use.

Fishhook Removal

The three basic methods of removing a fishhook are described below.

The push-through, snip-off method: As shown in figure 9, the steps are simple: A) Push the hook through. B) Snip it off. C) Back the barbless hook out. D) Treat the puncture wounds. While the technique seems straightforward, consider a few points: 1) Pushing the hook should not endanger underlying or adjacent structures. This limits the technique's usefulness, but it is still frequently an easy, quick method to employ. 2) Skin is not easy to push through. It is very elastic and will tent up over the barb as you try to push it through. Place side-cutting wire cutters, with jaws spread apart, over the point on the surface where you expect the hook point to punch through. 3) This is a painful process, and skin hurts when being poked from the bottom up, as much as from the top down. Once you start the procedure, get the push-through portion of this project over with in a hurry. 4) This adds a second puncture wound to the victim's anatomy. Cleanse the skin at the anticipated penetration site with soap or a surgical scrub before shoving the hook through. 5) When snipping off the protruding point, cover the wound area with your free hand to protect you and others from the flying hook point.

Figure 9
The push-through, snip-off method of removal

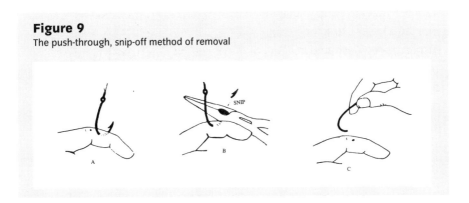

The string-jerk method: This works best in areas with little connective tissue. Fingers are loaded with fibrous tissue that tends to hinder a smooth hook removal. This technique works best in the back of the head, the shoulder, and most parts of the torso, arms, and legs. It is highly useful and can be virtually painless, causing minimal trauma.

First loop a line (such as the fish line) around the hook, ensuring that the line is held flush against the skin. Pushing down on the eye portion of the hook helps disengage the hook barb so that the quick pull will jerk the hook free with minimal trauma (see figure 10). Sometimes the hook is freed so fast that the victim doesn't realize the job has been completed!

The dissection method: This technique uses either a hypodermic needle or a sharp knife, and it should be reserved for instances of isolation with no hope of reaching professional help for several days.

Hooks that cannot be removed by the snip-off or string-jerk method should be taped in place, the fish line removed, and the patient evacuated to help. Avoid snipping off the hook near the skin surface, as this makes the physician's task of removal potentially more difficult. Place some triple-antibiotic ointment on the wound site twice daily until help can be reached.

Figure 10
The string-jerk method of fishhook removal

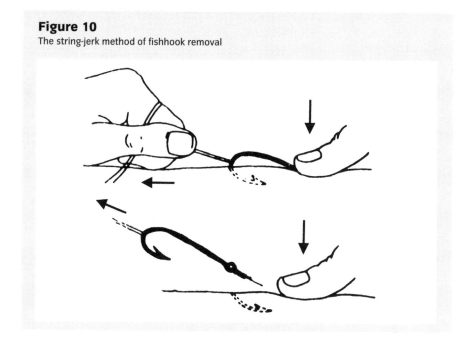

SPLINTER REMOVAL

Prepare the wound with surgical scrub, soapy water, or other cleansing solution that does not discolor the skin. Minute splinters are hard enough to see, and disguising them makes it even more difficult. If the splinter is shallow or the point buried, use a needle or sharp blade to tease the tissue over the splinter to remove this top layer. The splinter can then be pried out.

It is best to be aggressive and remove this top skin layer so that you can obtain a substantial bite on the splinter with the splinter forceps (or tweezers), rather than nibbling off the end of the splinter when making futile attempts to remove it with inadequate exposure. When using the splinter forceps, grasp the instrument between the thumb and forefinger, resting the instrument on the middle finger and further resting the entire hand against the victim's skin, if necessary, to prevent tremor. Approach the splinter from the side, if exposed, grasping it as low as possible. Apply triple-antibiotic ointment afterward.

If the wound was dirty, scrub afterward with Hibiclens or soapy water. If deep, treat as indicated above under puncture wounds with hot soaks and antibiotics.

CHAPTER EIGHT

Bone and Joint Injuries

(Sprains, Fractures, and Dislocations)

MANAGING ACUTE JOINT INJURIES— GENERAL PRINCIPLES

Proper care of joint injuries must be started immediately. Rest, ice, compression, and elevation form the basis of good first-aid management. Serious injuries with significant pain, swelling, or disfiguration will require treatment for shock (see page 7), stabilizing the injury with gentle support and light traction by hand, and then replacing hand traction with a splint. If there is angulation deformity of the limb—meaning the limb is at an angle at the site of the break—the injury should be straightened and the limb made to lie in the correct direction using gentle in-line traction prior to splint application. Cold should be applied for the first two days, as continuously as possible, but ensuring that a freezing injury does not occur. Afterward, applying heat for twenty minutes four times daily is helpful. Cold decreases the circulation, which lessens bleeding and swelling. Heat increases the circulation, which then aids the healing process. This technique applies to all injuries including muscle contusions and bruises.

Elevate the involved joint, if possible. Wrap with elastic bandage, or even strips of cloth, to immobilize the joint and provide moderate support once

Figure 11

Figure-eight technique of wrapping a support dressing around an ankle

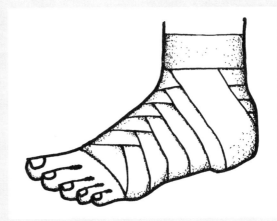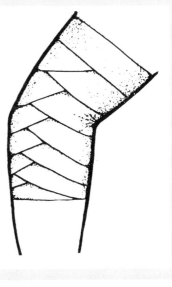

Figure 12

Figure-eight technique for supportive wrapping of the knee

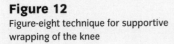

walking or use of the joint begins. Take care that the wrappings are not so tightly applied that they cut off the circulation.

Use crutches or other support to take enough weight off an injured ankle and knee to help decrease pain. The patient should not use an injured joint if use causes pain, as this indicates further strain on the already stressed ligaments or fracture. Conversely, if use of the injured part does not cause pain, additional damage is not being done, even if there is considerable swelling.

If the victim must walk on an injured ankle or knee, and doing so causes considerable pain, then support it the best way possible (wrapping, crutches, decreased carrying load, tight boot for ankle injury). Realize that further damage is being done, but that in your opinion the situation warrants such a sacrifice. Under emergency conditions a boot should not be removed from an injured ankle, as it may be difficult to replace it. However, one must avoid too much compression of the soft-tissue swelling to prevent circulation impairment. If the patient complains of increasingly severe pain, remove the boot. Also the boot should be removed within twenty-four hours of the injury, or sooner if the foot is wet. Remove the boot if the patient has decreased sensation in the foot or if there is a concern about possible cold injury.

Wrapping an ankle with an ace bandage is easy using the figure-eight technique as illustrated in figure 11. Simply wrap around the ankle, under and around the foot, and layer as shown.

Wrapping a knee is also performed using a figure-eight technique, as shown in figure 12. These wraps provide compression and slight support; however, they should never be applied so tightly that they cause discomfort or cut off circulation.

Pain medications may be given as needed, but elevation and decreased use will provide considerable pain relief for any bone or joint injury.

DISLOCATIONS

If the joint in question is deformed and/or the patient cannot move it, then the joint has suffered either a severe sprain or dislocation. Support the joint with sling or splint in such a manner that further stress is not applied to the joint.

The immediate reduction or replacement of shoulder, finger, kneecap, and nose dislocations can reduce pain and eliminate the necessity for an urgent evacuation. Replacement of other dislocations (ankle, knee, hip, and elbow particularly) aid in preventing circulation and nerve damage but still require urgent evacuation.

FRACTURES

"Fracture" is the medical term for a broken bone. At times it will be uncertain whether or not a fracture actually exists. If in doubt, splint and treat for pain, avoiding the use of the involved part. If the injury was simply a contusion, within a few days the pain will have diminished and the crisis may be over. If not, the likelihood of fracture is greater. In either case, a splint will provide the correct treatment.

TABLE 2—HOW TO SPLINT

Pad well.

Joint injury—immobilize bones above and below.

Bone injury—immobilize the joints above and below.

Broken bones, even significant contusions, will result in considerable swelling at the site of the injury. This deformity is made worse in the case of complete bone breaks, when the bone ends will usually ride over each other (or slip past each other), muscles will contract, and local bleeding will swell the tissues. Generally this swelling and deformity will cause no harm and should be treated by standard urban first-aid treatment, namely to splint the injury as it lies. However, the exception is the grossly angulated injury. When the wound has a significant angle (greater than 30 degrees), this causes potential harm in several ways. As the shortest distance between two points is a straight line, an angle in the wound means that the artery, vein, and nerve running alongside the bone are forced to go a longer distance. Whenever a hollow tube is stretched, the lumen, or center, is narrowed. This will result in a decrease in blood flow through these vessels. The nerve can also be harmed by the stretching trauma. Also some of the sharp pieces of bone will poke against the skin. No matter how well you pad the skin on the outside, these sharp pieces of bone might punch their way through the skin and create an open fracture, potentially resulting in a serious infection. For these reasons, grossly angulated fractures should be straightened by gentle in-line traction.

Before straightening a deformed limb, check the pulses beyond the fracture site. Compare the results of the injured side with the normal side of the victim. As the victim may be in mild shock, the pulses may be diminished on both sides. A more accurate method of checking the quality of blood flow is to check capillary filling. Do this by pressing down on the fingernail and suddenly releasing. Note the return of a flush of blood to the nail bed and, again, compare both sides to determine subtle differences in blood flow. Also check the nerve function. This is sometimes difficult and may even be impossible to perform. Ideally you are looking for decrease in grip strength or other muscle strength and numbness or radiating pain beyond the injury site. The severe pain of a fracture or serious contusion makes an accurate check of local nerve function very difficult to determine.

DIAGNOSING AND TREATING BONE AND JOINT INJURIES

Rather than discuss fractures and dislocations separately, it is best to discuss the body by region and thus look at diagnosis and treatment together.

Shoulder and Collarbone Injuries

Pain after trauma to a shoulder is due to a tendon or ligament injury, a broken bone, a joint separation, or even a dislocation. If the victim can use the shoulder, allow him to do it. Relieve pain with a sling for any injury in this area. A swath of cloth around the shoulder, holding the arm against the chest, gives maximal comfort but completely incapacitates the use of the shoulder. This is fine as long as the victim is not at risk of falling off an elevation or into water. In hazardous circumstances sling without a swath. An alternative to a sling and swath is to immobilize the shoulder by pinning a long-sleeve shirt arm to the chest with a safety pin or even buttoning the sleeve button to the opposite pocket buttonhole (see figure 13).

Figure 13
Two old U.S. Army techniques for immobilizing the shoulder

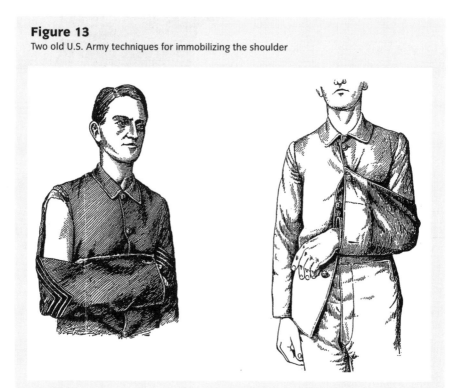

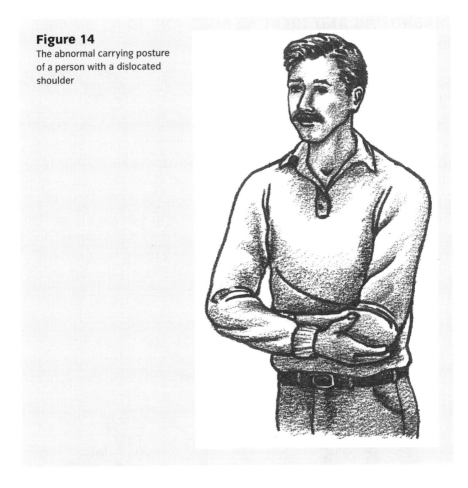

Figure 14
The abnormal carrying posture of a person with a dislocated shoulder

A shoulder dislocation requires immediate relocation to prevent nerve injury and terrible, debilitating pain. (Anterior dislocations of the shoulder joint account for more than 90 percent of shoulder dislocations. An anterior dislocation occurs when the top of the arm bone pops out of the socket and goes to the front.) The diagnosis of a shoulder dislocation is generally easy to make. The person cannot hold the injured arm against the chest wall, as he would be prone to do with any other serious injury of the upper arm (figure 14). As the arm is out of the socket, it cannot rotate down against the body. Not only is the arm held away from the body, but the normally round shoulder is flat.

A very easy but time-consuming method of putting the shoulder back in its socket is the Stimson maneuver. Have the patient lie on his stomach with the dislocated shoulder hanging toward the ground with ten to fifteen pounds

Figure 15
The Stimson technique for reducing shoulder dislocations

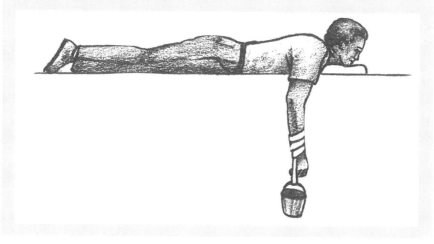

(five to seven kilograms) of weight secured to the hand (see figure 15). It usually takes at least twenty minutes for this method to work. The patient is aware of a sudden "clunk" as the shoulder relocates. While it is best to place the victim in a sling and swath for three weeks after this maneuver, the person can usually use the shoulder immediately to help self-evacuate.

Upper Arm Injuries

Fractures of the upper part of the arm (the top of the humerus) tend to be stable in older people. There is pain to touch in the upper arm, and eventually bruising becomes very noticeable in the lower part of the arm, forearm, and hand, but the person is usually willing to use the arm. If the break is not stable, he will not use the arm, as the pain from the fracture would be too great. A broken collarbone (clavicle) hurts too much to allow arm use. A sling and swath provide maximal pain relief. The classic splint is the figure-eight system, which holds the shoulders back, causing the bone fragments to be moved into a good position for healing. An empty backpack substitutes for this system very well. It is painful to have your shoulder pulled back when you have a broken collarbone. A sling and swath on the injured side provide additional pain relief, but the victim will probably have to sleep sitting up, as attempting to lie flat will move the broken bone and increase the pain unbearably.

Pain at the middle of the upper arm can mean a break or serious contusion.

In either case, immobilize the arm against the chest wall with a sling and swath. If it is a severe, unstable break, it will also require a padded splint.

Elbow Injuries

Injuries of the elbow should be splinted incorporating the upper and lower arm. Splint the victim as you found him, but do not keep the elbow in a 90-degree position; allow the joint to droop open. This reduces pressure that the bleeding might cause in the front of the elbow, which in turn could result in decreased blood flow to the rest of the arm.

Forearm Injuries

Possible fractures of the forearm should be splinted to include the elbow and wrist. If possible, splint the elbow with 80 to 90 degrees of bend to elevate the forearm and hand and reduce swelling.

Apply a rigid splint, such as the Sam Splint. Splint fractures of the forearm with the hand placed in the position of function (the relaxed, curled position that you would normally hold your hand in while walking; see figure 16). Place a rolled-up sock, glove, or other soft material into the palm and immobilize the hand, wrist, and forearm in a splint. Encourage exercise of the hand to aid circulation.

Correct marked angulation as mentioned on page 27. Gentle traction results in an overall improvement of circulation with a negligible risk of creating further blood vessel or nerve damage. Move slowly and stop if force is required for further movement or if the patient complains of significantly increasing pain.

Wrist Injuries

Fractures, dislocations, and sprains of the wrist can all be splinted with a rigid splint such as the Sam Splint. If circulation to the hand is decreased by significant deformity, apply gentle in-line traction to improve the position.

Hand/Finger Injuries

Deformity and limited motion is an indication of a dislocation. Replace dislocated fingers by placing the joint into a slight bend, applying traction, and pushing the protruding part back into position. Try to correct the deformity immediately, as the pain increases and becomes difficult to lessen. Soaking in cold water or applying an ice pack will help with swelling. Dislocations of the base of the thumb and index finger are very difficult to replace. After one attempt, immobilize in the slightly curved position of function.

Figure 16
Sam Splint Splinting Techniques

The Sam Splint is a foam-padded, malleable aluminum strip that can be easily molded into various splints, as illustrated. Forming a slight ridge by pinching the metal makes the aluminum strip rigid.

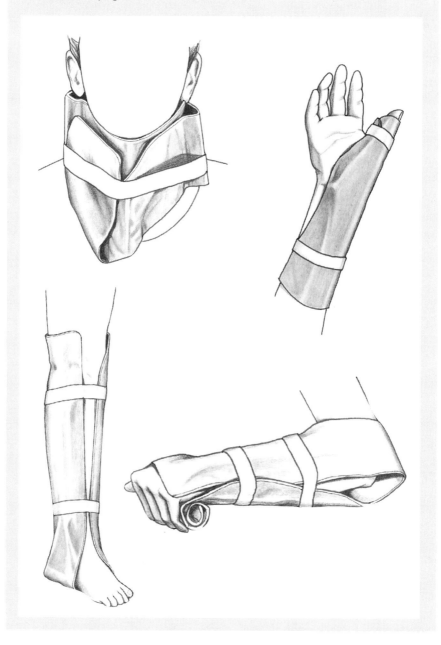

Deformities or point tenderness not associated with the joints is probably due to a fracture, and angulation certainly is. Immediately attempt to straighten the deformity. A Sam Splint can be cut to fit the finger. Never splint an injured finger in a straight position, but always curve it into the position of function.

Hip Dislocation and Fracture

If a patient has had significant injury, pain when standing, and very painful motion in the region of the hip, carry him out on a litter. Secure the leg on the injured side to the uninjured leg. Try to avoid placing possible fractures of the hip in traction.

Figure 17 demonstrates typical posturing found in people with anterior and posterior hip dislocation and a fractured thigh bone (femur). While this positioning is not absolute, it provides a strong clue to the diagnosis. Dislocations of either type are difficult to splint as the patient resists placing the hip into a neutral position.

Figure 17

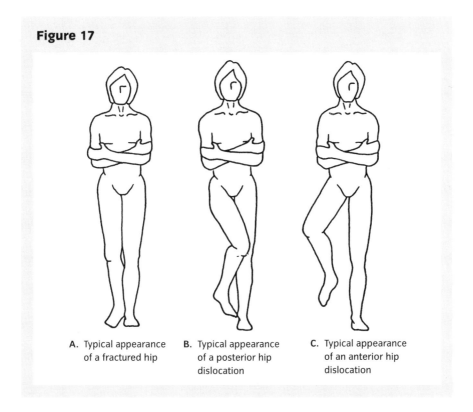

A. Typical appearance of a fractured hip

B. Typical appearance of a posterior hip dislocation

C. Typical appearance of an anterior hip dislocation

These injuries are very serious. Tremendous blood loss occurs internally. Fractures of the hip cause pain in the anterior media aspect (front and side) of the thigh. Dislocations in younger people may be associated with fractures; in older people fractures are common and are the probable cause of the deformity.

Posterior dislocation of the hip (rather than central fracture-dislocations and anterior hip dislocations) is more common in healthy young adults. All of these injuries are infrequent when compared, for instance, with dislocation of the shoulder. Posterior dislocations can cause injury to the sciatic nerve, the main nerve of the leg. This can cause shooting pains down the back of the leg and/or numbness of the lower leg. It is most important that reduction of the dislocation not be delayed more than twenty-four hours. Muscle relaxation and pain medication will be needed. To reduce pain, place the victim on his back with the knee and hip in a 90-degree position—the line of the femur pointing vertically upward. The thigh should be pulled steadily upward while the femur is simultaneously rotated externally.

For evacuation purposes, pad the leg well and buddy-splint the injured leg to the other leg. This victim will require a litter. Continued pressure on, or severe injury to, the sciatic nerve will cause muscle wasting and loss of sensation to practically the whole leg. This damage must be surgically repaired as soon as possible; in the extreme case of survival without possible repair, brace the affected leg to allow mobility by the victim and care for the numb skin areas to prevent sores and infection.

Central fracture/dislocations result when the head of the femur is driven through the socket into the pelvis. Light traction can be applied for comfort by means of adhesive tape applied to the lower leg. Anterior dislocation results from forceful injuries, such as airplane crashes and motorcycle accidents. An examination of the lower leg demonstrates considerable lateral rotation or outward tilting of the foot when the victim is lying on his back. Reduction of the anterior hip dislocation is as described under posterior dislocation with traction on the flexed limb, but combine with medial rotation—or rotating the limb inward rather than outward.

Thighbone Fracture

Fractures of the femur can, of course, occur from the hip to the knee. They are classified and treated by orthopedic specialists differently according to the location of the break.

The first-aid treatment consists of treating for shock and immobilizing the limb, initially using a traction splint. Start by providing pain relief with gentle hands on in-line traction (see page 27). Then rig a trucker's hitch or, weather permitting, tape directly to the skin to form the traction splint as illustrated in figure 18.

Figure 18
Trucker's hitch

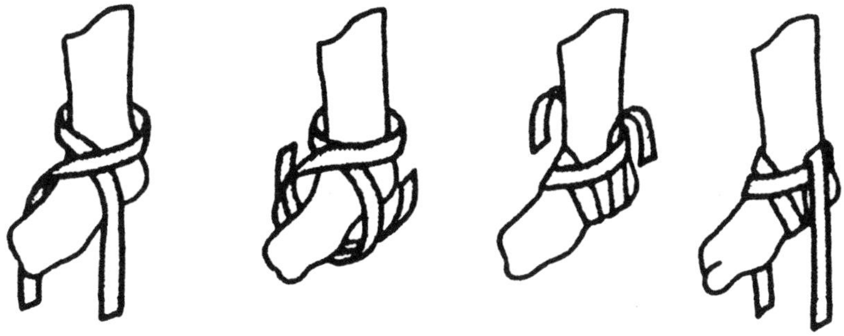

Traction splinting is initially required because spasms from the powerful muscles in this region cause considerable overriding of bone fragments, increasing the extent of the injury. Traction also reestablishes the normal length and configuration of the musculature and tightens the membranes that surround the muscle (the fascia); this tends to decrease the bleeding that occurs with this injury. Additionally the application of a proper traction splint can result in significant pain reduction. During prolonged transport the patient can be comfortably removed from the traction splint periodically. After several days she may do quite well with a buddy-splint to the other leg during litter transport. Prolonged use of the trucker's hitch traction splint system can lead to necrosis—or death—of the skin of the ankle due to the constant pressure.

Dislocated Kneecap

The kneecap (patella) usually dislocates laterally—to the outside of the knee. This dislocation results in a locking of the knee, and the bump to one side makes the diagnosis obvious. Relocate the patella by flexing the hip and the knee. When straightening the knee the patella usually snaps back into place by itself. If not, just push it back into place while straightening the knee on the next try. Splint with a tube splint (Ensolite foam), with the knee slightly flexed. This patient should be able to walk.

Knee Sprains/Dislocations/Fractures

If pain in the knee is severe, then several diagnoses are possible. There may be tears of ligaments, tendon, or cartilage. Or there may be associated dislocations or fractures. All you really can assess is the amount of pain that the patient is having, and you have to take his word for that. The amount of swelling or deformity will give you a clue, but the most important aspect of care will be determined by the pain level relayed to you by the patient.

Have the patient lie as comfortably as possible. Rest, Ice, Compress, Elevate (RICE) the knee. In case of significant pain and/or swelling, remove the boot (depending on the weather) and check the pulse on top of the foot (the dorsal pedal pulse); question the victim about sensation in the feet. Check the dorsal pedal pulse on the opposite side for comparison. If the injury appears minor, this check is not necessary.

Significant deformity means that a dislocation may have occurred. Serious disruption of the blood vessels and nerve damage can take place. Check for pulse and sensation in the foot. If these are all right, splint the knee as it lies. If not, have a helper hold the lower thigh while you grip the ankle with one hand and the calf with the other. Use in-line traction while you gently flex the knee to see if you can reposition it better. If the pain is too great, you meet resistance, or you cannot do it, splint in the most comfortable position and evacuate as soon as possible.

Even without obvious deformity an immediate complaint, or continuing complaint, about significant pain means that you now have a litter case and you should make plans accordingly. If in two hours, the next morning, or two days later, the patient feels better and wishes to walk on it—great! Let him. You should remove all weight from his shoulders and provide him with a cane. Have him use the cane on the side opposite the injury. This places a more natural force vector on the injured joint. And continue the compressive dressing. After two days begin applying heat packs during rest stops and in the evening. The patient's perception of pain should be the key to managing these injuries in the bush.

Ankle Sprains/Dislocations/Fractures

Generally fractures of both sides of the ankle are associated with a dislocation. The severe pain associated with the fractures will be an early indication that this patient is a litter case. Splint the ankle with a single Sam Splint or form a trough of Ensolite foam and tape it on. The latter is not a walking splint, but if the pain is significant enough, the patient will not be walking anyway. A flail ankle, caused by complete disruption of the ankle ligaments, readily slops back into position and can be held in place with a trough splint of Ensolite padding.

Allow the patient to rest after the injury before attempting to walk. If there is severe pain, it might be broken or badly sprained. Either way, if the pain is too severe, that patient will not be walking, at least not until the pain subsides. As with the knee, if the pain diminishes enough that the victim can walk, allow him to do so with a cane and no extra weight.

Foot Injuries

Stubbed toes can be buddy-splinted to provide pain relief. If they have been stubbed to the extent that they deviate at a crazy angle sideways, they should be repositioned before buddy-splint. Place a pencil (or an object of similar width) on the side opposite the bend and use it as a fulcrum to help snap the toe back into alignment.

The pain caused by the pressure due to bleeding under a toenail can be relieved by draining it through a hole bored in the nail with a sharp object.

Severe pain in the arch of the foot or in the metatarsals (the bones between the ankle and toes) can represent fractures or sprains. RICE as described on page 36. Staying off the foot for a short time might reduce pain in minor injuries, but it takes weeks for a fracture to decrease in severity. Lighten the patient's weight load and provide a cane. If the foot swells to the extent that the boot cannot be placed on the foot, consider cutting the boot along the sides and taping it onto the foot. This provides support for the foot and ankle.

CHAPTER NINE

Head Injuries

Not all head injuries require immediate evacuation. If there has been a relatively trivial injury—no loss of consciousness or a loss of consciousness for less than thirty seconds before returning to a full normal alertness—in patients with no history of a bleeding disorder and not on medications that might increase the risk of bleeding (such as aspirin), monitor for twenty-four hours and awaken every two hours for evaluation. Watch for: 1) changes in mental status, including personality changes, lethargy, drowsiness, disorientation, unusual irritability, and combativeness; 2) persistent nausea and vomiting; 3) loss of visual acuity; and 4) alterations in coordination and/or speech. If these signs or symptoms appear, then an evacuation should be initiated.

Immediate evacuation is recommended for all patients who have received a blow to the head or face that results in loss of consciousness for more than two minutes or who have:

- Debilitating headache
- Alterations in mental status (see above)
- Persistent nausea and vomiting
- Bruising behind and below the ears
- Bruising around the eyes
- Loss of coordination
- Even partial loss of vision
- Appearance of clear fluid (possibly cerebral spinal fluid) from the nose
- Seizures
- Relapses into unconsciousness

If there is an obvious head injury, consider the possibility of a neck injury (see chapter 10).

During the evacuation maintain the airway by keeping the patient in a stable side position, which also helps prevent the possibility of inhaling vomit, a common threat with head-injured patients. While all persons with head injuries are strapped to a backboard in an urban setting, this is not necessary if the patient assessment does not indicate that evacuation is required. When the evacuation is started, a reassessment of the requirements for neck or spine immobilization should be made periodically. If the spine can be cleared, rigid immobilization should be terminated, even though the evacuation process is continued.

CHAPTER TEN

Neck and Back Injury Management

In the city many patients placed in full spinal immobilization will prove not to have unstable spine injuries, but this precaution will protect the few who do. In the wilderness, full spinal immobilization may present unnecessary hardship and danger to both patients and rescuers. The challenge is to seek a balance between the difficulties and dangers of evacuating an immobilized patient versus not immobilizing a spinal injury.

CLEARING THE SPINE

To evacuate more easily and rapidly from an area of immediate danger, it may be safer for the patient and rescuers to omit spinal immobilization—or to use only partial spinal immobilization, such as a cervical collar. All patients with signs or symptoms of spinal injury, however, should be immobilized. This would include persons with neck pain (not just tightness), point tenderness to touch along the spine, numbness or tingling or pain radiating into an arm or leg, or any pain in the neck while she gently moves her neck through a range of motion (with adequate handheld head support for safety).

Patients with no signs or symptoms need not be immobilized despite significant accident, unless they have other injuries or show any signs of impaired mental function. If at any point the patient begins to complain of pain, weakness, or numbness, immobilize the spine.

IMMOBILIZING THE SPINE

Treatment consists of full immobilization in a rigid litter or immobilization on the most level ground available with a cervical collar until a rigid litter can be improvised or brought in. Once again, if at any point the patient begins to complain of pain, you should immobilize the spine.

A cervical collar can be built with a Sam Splint as indicated in figure 16. It may be improvised by placing sandbags on either side of the neck while the patient is still on the ground. If the victim is lying twisted around debris and in a dangerous location, she will have to be moved. The head will need to be supported by gentle hand traction, with the head and neck stabilized by one person, who will direct the actions of others helping to move the patient. The technique is called a "log roll" and is used to help examine the patient and to move her onto insulation or a stretcher.

The Log Roll

Ideally several people will work together to logroll a patient. The rescuers station themselves along the same side of the patient with one person facing them at the head of the patient. This person will assume the role of directing all movements of the group and will provide hand stabilization to the patient's head and neck. Place the patient's hands along her sides. The rescuers reach across the patient at the shoulder, hip, and upper and lower legs and roll the victim toward themselves on the command of the "head" rescuer. The back of the patient is visually examined and adequate insulation or a rigid stretcher can be placed alongside the victim. On command the rescuers roll the victim upon the stretcher. Always fabricate a neck collar to provide some protection and to remind the patient not to move the neck. When the professional rescuers arrive, they will direct packaging the patient to prevent further neck and spine injury. In the meantime, prevent movement of the patient by placing padded rocks, socks filled with sand, or otherwise surrounding the patient with a packing of clothing or soft articles.

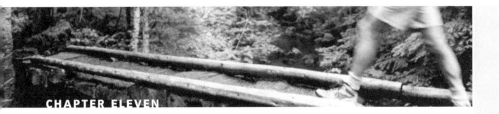

CHAPTER ELEVEN

Eye

Eye problems in the wilderness can range from irritations from smoke and insect repellent, abrasions from foliage, flying embers striking the eye, allergies, ultraviolet damage from snow or water reflection (snow blindness), eye infection, foreign body, and contact lens problems to blunt or sharp injuries to the eye surface or deeper tissues.

SMOKE OR INSECT REPELLENT IRRITATIONS

In the sometimes desperate attempt to avoid insects, nearly all woodspersons find themselves sooner or later resorting to standing near a smoky fire or using DEET insect repellent to keep bugs at bay. However, both methods can cause eye irritation. The wilderness treatment is simple. Rinse the eyes with eyewash or clean water. And do not rub them!

FOREIGN BODY IN EYE

Carefully shine a small light at the surface of the eye from one side to see if a minute speck becomes visible. By moving the light back and forth, you might see movement of a shadow on the iris of the eye and thus confirm the presence of a foreign body. A shadow that consistently stays put with blinking is probably a foreign body.

When examining an eye for a foreign body, also be sure to check under the eyelid. Turn the upper lid outward over a Q-tip swab, thus examining not only the eyeball but also the undersurface of the eyelid. Remove the foreign body by blinking with the eye submerged in water or by gentle prodding with the moist end of a folded piece of cloth.

THE EYE PATCH

You should patch an eye for pain relief and protection (figure 19). Severe injuries may require patching both eyes to minimize the blink reflex.

TABLE 3—PATCHING SUPPLIES

Strips of tape

Simple pad of cloth/gauze

Ring of cloth

Figure 19
Eye patch serious injuries with a ring of cloth.

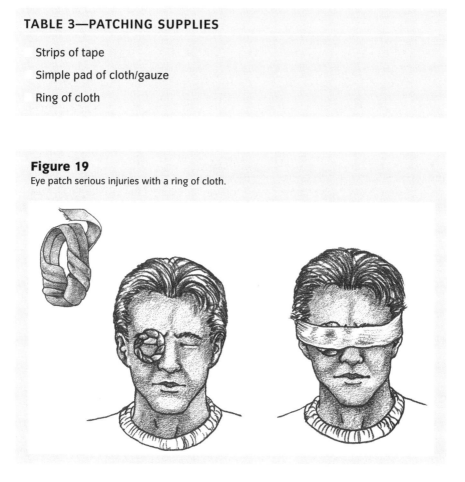

EYE ABRASION

Examine the eye surface carefully to ensure that no foreign body is present. Check under the eyelids as discussed above. An abrasion on the eye will feel like a foreign body is present. Treat with soothing eyedrops if available, or place a cold, damp cloth on the eye. Even a damp cloth will provide some relief due to evaporative cooling. Patch for comfort as indicated above.

PINK EYE

Irritation from any source will cause the white of the eye to become "pink." A pink eye can therefore indicate a bacterial or viral infection, allergy, or irritation. Ensure that the cause is not due to a foreign body and, if it is, treat as indicated above. Eyes irritated by a foreign body or trauma, such as an abrasion, will feel better if patched. Eyes irritated from allergies or infection do not require patching, but the patient will feel better with both eyes protected from bright light by the use of sunglasses. As a temporary measure various soothing eyedrops and ointments are available without prescription, or rinse the eye with clean water frequently during the day. If nasal congestion is also present, treatment with a decongestant and antihistamine is quite appropriate.
Return to civilization for medical evaluation.

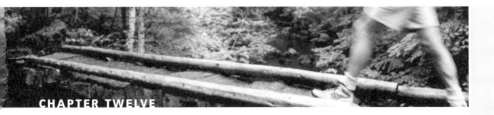

CHAPTER TWELVE

Ear

Pulling on the earlobe will elicit pain in swimmer's ear. This will not hurt if the patient has a middle-ear infection. A history of head congestion can also indicate middle-ear infection.

SWIMMER'S EAR

The external ear canal generally becomes inflamed from conditions of high humidity, accumulation of earwax, or contact with contaminated water. Scratching the ear after touching the nose or scratching elsewhere may also help transmit this common infection.

Treatment: Prevent cold air from blowing against the ear. Applying warm packs against the ear or instilling comfortably warm sweet oil, or even clean cooking oil, can help. Provide pain medication. **Return** for medical help if the patient develops a fever, the pain becomes severe, or lymph nodes or adjacent neck tissues start swelling.

MIDDLE-EAR INFECTION

This condition may appear in a person who has sinus congestion and possibly results from drainage due to allergy or infection. The ear pain can be excruciating. Fever will frequently be intermittent, normal at one moment and over 103°F (39°C) at other times. If the eardrum ruptures, the pain will cease immediately and the fever will drop. This drainage allows the body to cure the infection but will result in at least temporary damage to the eardrum and decreased hearing until it heals.

Treatment: Provide decongestant, pain medication, and oral prescription antibiotic. Give oral pain medication. **Return** for professional treatment.

FOREIGN BODY IN THE EAR

There are three types of foreign bodies that end up in ears: accumulation of wax plugs, foreign objects, and live insects.

Treatment: Wax plugs can usually be softened with warmed oil. This may have to be placed in the ear canal repeatedly over many days. Irrigating with room temperature water may be attempted with a bulb syringe. If a wax-plugged ear becomes painful, treat as indicated in the section on swimmer's ear. Attempt to grasp a foreign body with a pair of tweezers only if you can see it. Irrigation may be attempted as discussed above. Drown an insect with cooking oil, then attempt removal. Oil seems to kill bugs quicker than water. The less struggle, the less chance for stinging, biting, or other trauma to the delicate ear canal and eardrum. Tilt the ear downward, to assist in sliding the dead bug toward the entrance, where it can be grasped. Shining a light at the ear to coax a bug out is probably futile. **Return** for treatment if the problem becomes painful.

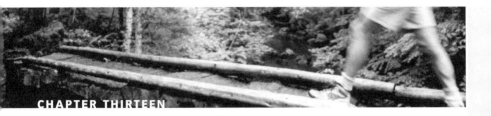

CHAPTER THIRTEEN

Nose

FOREIGN BODY IN THE NOSE

Foul drainage from one nostril may well indicate a foreign body. In a child drainage from one nostril must be considered to be a foreign body until ruled out.

Treatment: Have the patient try to blow his nose to remove the foreign body. With an infant it may be possible for a parent to gently puff into the baby's mouth to force the object out of the nose. Stretch the nostril open with a blunt-tipped tweezer. One can stretch the nostril quite extensively without causing pain. Shine a light into the nostril passage and attempt to spot the foreign body. Try to grasp the object with forceps or other instrument while within your sights. After removing a foreign body, be sure to check the nostril again for an additional one. Try not to push a foreign body down the back of the patient's throat where he may choke on it. If this is unavoidable, have the patient face down and bend over to decrease the chance of choking.

NOSEBLEED

If nosebleeding is caused from a contusion to the nose, the bleeding is usually brisk but stops on its own. Bleeding that starts without trauma is generally more difficult to stop. Most bleeding is from small arteries located near the front of the nose partition, or nasal septum.

Treatment: Use direct pressure. Have the victim squeeze the nose between his fingers for ten minutes by the clock, squashing the soft area beneath the hard bone of the nose. If this fails, squeeze another ten minutes. Do not blow the nose, for this will dislodge clots and start the bleeding all over again. If the bleeding is severe, have the victim sit up to aid in the reduction of the blood pressure in the nose and lean forward to prevent choking on blood. **Evacuate** if bleeding cannot be stopped.

CHAPTER FOURTEEN

Teeth/Mouth

CAVITIES

A visual examination or gentle tapping on the suspect tooth may identify cavities.

Treatment: Dry the tooth and try to clean out any cavity you find. For many years oil of cloves, or eugenol, has been used to deaden dental pain. Do not apply an aspirin directly to a painful tooth; it will only make things worse. A daub of topical anesthetic such as 1 percent dibucaine ointment will help deaden dental pain. And, of course, give pain medication if you have any.

LOOSE TOOTH

Treatment: When you examine a traumatized mouth and find a tooth that is rotated or dislocated in any direction, do not push the tooth back into place. Further movement may disrupt the tooth's blood and nerve supply. If the tooth is at all secure, leave it alone. The musculature of the lips and tongue will generally gently push the tooth back into place and keep it there.

BROKEN TOOTH

Treatment: A fractured tooth with exposed pink substance that is bleeding is showing exposed nerve. This tooth will need protection with eugenol as indicated above. **Evacuate:** This is actually a dental emergency that should be treated by a dentist immediately.

LOST TOOTH

Treatment: If a tooth is knocked out, replace it into the socket immediately. If this cannot be done, have the victim hold the tooth under her tongue or in her lower lip until it can be implanted. **Evacuate:** Hours are a matter of great importance. A tooth left out too long will be rejected by the body as a foreign substance.

MOUTH LACERATION

Cuts in the tongue or mouth will initially bleed profusely.

Treatment: Pack a clean piece of cloth against the open area to staunch the bleeding. Seldom are stitches required to close these wounds. After the bleeding has been controlled, rinse the mouth with a dilute saltwater swish every two hours. **Return:** A physician should see the patient, but evacuation is not urgent.

CHAPTER FIFTEEN

Abdominal Problems

Pain in the abdominal area can range from minor to severe, from a passing nuisance to a fatal situation. Making the correct diagnosis and providing the correct treatment can be one of the greatest challenges of medicine, especially when you are in the wilderness.

Evacuate 1) if the patient seems to be getting worse after a hour; 2) if he becomes lightheaded when standing; 3) when he has a rapid pulse rate (certainly over 110) when lying down; or 4) if there is progressive weakness, intractable vomiting and/or diarrhea, an inability to tolerate oral fluids. Professional help should also be sought if fever persists longer than twenty-four hours.

NAUSEA AND VOMITING

Nausea and vomiting are frequently caused by infections known as gastroenteritis. Many times these are viral, so that an antibiotic is of no value. These infections will usually resolve themselves without treatment in twenty-four to forty-eight hours. Fever seldom is high, but it may briefly be high in some cases. Fever should not persist above 100°F longer than twelve hours.

Treatment of fever and discomfort is best accomplished with acetaminophen rather than aspirin or ibuprofen, which may cause further stomach irritation. Use antacid and meclizine if available.

HEARTBURN

Gastritis, ulcer, and hiatal hernia (which is a cause of stomach acid reflux) all cause a burning sensation in the upper portion of the stomach. In the case of reflux, the burning pain radiates into the center of the chest.

Treatment: Use an antacid to neutralize the acid burn and to help prevent further damage. If you have no antacid handy, try eating food to absorb the acid. Avoid any food with tomato products, spicy foods, and acidic foods.

MOTION SICKNESS

Motion sickness may be avoided by staring at the far horizon and not at nearby objects.

Treatment: To prevent and treat motion sickness, a very useful nonprescription drug is meclizine 25 mg, taken one hour prior to departure for all-day protection. If vomiting occurs, replace fluids as indicated below.

DIARRHEA

Diarrhea is the expulsion of watery stool. This malady usually stops on its own but can be a threat to life, depending upon its cause and extent. The most frequent cause of diarrhea is infection. And the infection normally comes from poor hygiene (for example, not washing eating utensils well enough) or from a dirty water supply.

Treatment: Prevent dehydration. Fluid replacement needs to be encouraged, even though the person feels like the fluid is just running right through him. Provide the patient with an amount of fluid equal to the diarrhea volume, plus at least 3 quarts (2.8 liters) daily. It is essential to keep up with the fluid loss. Adults will do fine with plain water, but children or debilitated people should use oral rehydration/electrolyte solutions (ORS).

TABLE 4—HOMEMADE ORS

Use alternating glasses of:

- Glass #1: 8 oz. (230 ml) fruit juice (such as apple, orange, or lemon); ½ teaspoon (2.5 ml) honey or corn syrup; and 1 pinch salt
- Glass #2: 8 oz. (230 ml) water (boiled or treated) and ¼ teaspoon (1.2 ml) baking soda

Plain salt and sugar solutions, similar to those used for heat/exercise replacement, can be used for mild dehydration but are not adequate for serious dehydration or replacement of continuing high losses. For mild dehydration, partial maintenance, or supplementation, or where nothing else is available, rice water, fruit juice, coconut milk, or diluted cola drinks may suffice.

WATER PURIFICATION

Water can be purified adequately for drinking by mechanical, physical, and chemical means. Chlorine-based systems are very effective against virus and bacteria. They work best in neutral or slightly acid waters. Iodine is also effective and is not as affected by water acid or alkali content. The chemical purification techniques are easy to use, cheap, and generally effective, thus ensuring their popularity. However, neither of these chemical systems works well against parasitic types of waterborne infection such as giardia, cryptosporidium, and other similar wilderness parasites. A new chemical flocculation system is the ideal chemical system, as it will also eliminate all of the resistant parasites.

Filtration systems provide effective means of removing parasites and bacteria depending upon the type, eliminating contamination from chemical pollutants. High-quality porcelain systems (such as the Katadyn) or combination filter/chemical systems also eliminate viruses.

Figure 20
A solar still condenses drinkable water from vegetation or contaminated sources. It is very slow and produces only minimal amounts of water.

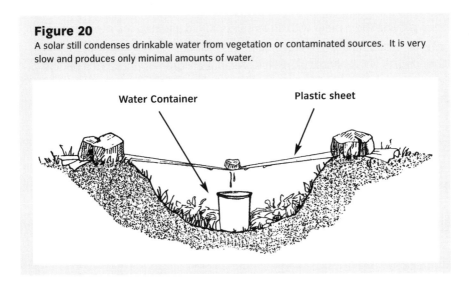

Water Container   Plastic sheet

Another method of water purification has been with us a long time—fire. Bringing water to a boil will effectively kill pathogens and make water safe to drink, even at high altitudes. Simply bringing water to 150°F (65.5°C) is adequate to kill the pathogens discussed above, and all others besides. At high altitude the boiling point of water is reduced. For example, at 25,000 feet the boiling point of water would be about 185°F (85°C)—still adequate to do the job!

Water may be obtained by squeezing any freshwater fish and from some plants. Never drink urine or seawater, as the high solute content of these liquids will only dehydrate you more and make the problem worse. A solar still can be prepared for reprocessing urine, water from grass, etc., as indicated in figure 20. In water-poor areas, catching rainwater may be an essential part of routine survival. Be careful of melting ice: Treat all ice-melt water as indicated above, because there is a very strong chance that ice deposits are contaminated.

CHAPTER SIXTEEN

High-Altitude Illness

Traveling from lower regions to above 1 mile of elevation will frequently cause headache, nausea, and other symptoms similar to mild flu. In fact a whole cluster of symptoms may make the unwary high-country traveler very uncomfortable. The most common of these problems are acute mountain sickness (AMS), high-altitude pulmonary edema (HAPE), high-altitude cerebral edema (HACE), and peripheral edema.

Limiting the rate of ascent can prevent people's becoming ill from altitude. Get used to the altitude slowly by gradually increasing the altitude of overnight camps. The first camp should be no higher than 8,000 feet (2,400 meters), with an increase of no more than 1,000 to 2,000 feet (300 to 600 meters) per night. Otherwise spend two nights at the same altitude for every 2,000-foot (600-meter) gain in altitude above 10,000 feet (3,000 meters). When a trip is started at over 9,000 feet (2,700 meters), two nights should be spent acclimatizing at that altitude before proceeding higher. Always attempt to sleep at the lowest elevation possible (climb high, sleep low).

Other methods of preventing high-altitude illness include a high-carbohydrate diet, moderate exercise to avoid excessive fatigue and shortness of breath, proper hydration, and the use of certain prophylactic medications under a doctor's supervision. The drugs commonly used are acetazolamide and dexamethasone. Acetazolamide is considered the drug of choice for chemical prevention of AMS.

Treatment: "Descent, descent, descent" is the treatment for all forms of high-altitude illness. However, mild forms of altitude illness usually resolve spontaneously in two to four days and descent is not necessary. Note that all ill persons must not be left alone or sent down alone.

ACUTE MOUNTAIN SICKNESS (AMS)

The symptoms of acute mountain sickness (AMS) include headache, loss of appetite, nausea, insomnia, decreased urination, and fatigue, basically resembling an alcohol hangover.

Treatment/Return: Descend or at least stop further ascent and wait for improvement before proceeding. Use pain and nausea medication as necessary. Prescription therapy includes giving acetazolamide 250 mg twice daily. If the illness progresses, descent is mandatory.

HIGH-ALTITUDE PULMONARY EDEMA (HAPE)

This problem is rare below 8,000 feet (2,500 meters). Mild HAPE symptoms are decreased exercise performance, fatigue, shortness of breath during exertion but not at rest, a dry cough, and localized chest congestion. In moderate to severe HAPE there is marked weakness and fatigue, blue discoloration of the lips and fingernail beds, and a dry to raspy cough. If it progresses the cough becomes productive, and a gurgling sensation or sound forms in the chest. The diagnosis of HAPE is certain if there is a breathing rate of twenty breaths per minute or a heart rate greater than 130 beats per minute after twenty minutes of rest.

Treatment/Evacuate: Immediate descent is essential in moderate to severe cases, with 2,000 to 4,000 feet (600 to 1,200 meters) usually being sufficient. Keep the patient warm and exert the patient as little as possible. Advanced treatment consists of oxygen and the prescription drugs acetazolamide 250 mg twice daily and nifedipine 60 mg every six hours. A portable hyperbaric chamber (Gamow Bag) is highly useful in reversing the effects of high altitude and can make a nonambulatory patient ambulatory. Descent after treatment by either the Gamow Bag or the medical therapies is still essential.

HIGH-ALTITUDE CEREBRAL EDEMA (HACE)

Death has occurred from HACE at altitudes as low as 8,000 feet (2,500 meters), but it is rare below 11,500 feet (3,500 meters). HACE is a continuation of the brain swelling that causes AMS, but at this point the swelling has progressed to the point that it has become dangerous and will kill the patient if descent is not immediate. Symptoms include progressive neurological deterioration, with changes in consciousness and loss of coordination, accompanied by impaired judgment, hallucinations, severe headache, and eventually coma. When the coma develops, the patient usually dies within twelve hours. The best diagnostic clue to HACE is the patient's inability to walk a straight 30-foot line.

Treatment/Evacuate: Descent is the critical and most important therapy for these patients. Other medical treatments include high-flow oxygen, injections of dexamathasone, and the Gamow Bag.

CHAPTER SEVENTEEN

Cold and Heat Injuries

Exposure to either hot or cold temperatures can result in severe injuries, even death, if not managed appropriately. Proper clothing, head protection, physical fitness, prevention of exhaustion, nutrition, and adequate water intake are essential to prevent injury in hot or cold environments.

HYPOTHERMIA

The term "hypothermia" refers to the lowering of the body's core temperature to 95°F (35°C) while "profound hypothermia" is a core temperature lower than 90°F (32°C). Hypothermia can occur quickly when exposed to cold water (acute hypothermia) or more slowly from cold-weather exposure (chronic hypothermia). Hypothermia is the most likely of the environmental injuries encountered in the outdoors. Most chronic hypothermia deaths occur when the temperature is between 30°F (− 1°C) and 50°F (10°C). There is increased risk of acute hypothermia when the sum of the air and water temperature adds up to less than 100°F (43°C).

Chronic exposure hypothermia will soon develop in anyone who becomes exhausted. A tired person will not be able to work hard and produce as much heat. Taking temperatures in the field is difficult, primarily because oral readings can be inaccurate and rectal temperatures expose the victim to further cooling and are usually impractical. Detection of chronic hypothermia is made by two observations. The first is violent shivering. Shivering, however, will stop when the person becomes exhausted or the muscle temperature cools to 86°F

(30°C). The second is loss of coordination. A person who cannot walk a straight 30-foot (9-meter) line is hypothermic.

Be suspicious that someone is ill from acute hypothermia when she has been in cold water for longer than twenty minutes.

Treatment: Prevent further heat loss, provide food and fluid, and allow the patient to rest covered with adequate insulation. If the patient is shivering, there will be an internal heat production that results in rewarming. If you apply heat to the skin with hot packs or cuddling, you may extinguish the shivering response and actually slow the rewarming. If the patient is incapable of shivering because of exhaustion or profound cold muscle, adding heat will be inadequate to rewarm her in the field. **Evacuate** persons who are incapable of rewarming. If evacuation is not possible, place two rescuers in two sleeping bags zipped together with the victim. Keep everyone's head within the bag system to allow the victim to rebreathe the rescuers' expired air. This adds little heat, but it does place this small amount in an important core location.

FROSTBITE

Frostbite is the freezing of tissue. Outside temperatures must be below freezing for frostbite to occur; in fact skin temperature must be cooled to between 22°F to 24°F (-5.5°C to -4.4°C) before tissue will freeze. The underlying physical condition of the victim, length of cold contact, and type of cold contact (such as cold metal or fuel) are other important factors leading to frostbite.

Deep frostbite flesh will not indent when pressed upon, while superficial frostbite flesh will also be waxy colored and cold and will indent.

Treatment: When superficial frostbite is suspected, thaw immediately so that it does not become a more serious, deep frostbite. Warm the hands by withdrawing them into the victim's coat through the sleeves—avoid opening the front of the coat to minimize heat loss. Feet should be thawed against a companion or cupped in your own hands in a roomy sleeping bag or otherwise in an insulated environment. NEVER, NEVER rub snow on a frostbitten area. For victims with deep frostbite, rapid rewarming in 110°F (43°C) water is the most effective treatment. This thawing may take twenty to thirty minutes, but it should be continued until all paleness at the tips of the fingers or toes has turned pink or burgundy red—and then stopped. This will be very painful and will require pain medication. Refreezing would result in substantial tissue loss. Also once the victim has been thawed, very careful management of the thawed part is required. The patient will need a stretcher if the foot is involved. Tissue damage increases with the length of time that it is allowed to remain frozen.

IMMERSION FOOT

It is essential that anyone going into the outdoors knows how to prevent this injury. It results from wet, cool conditions with temperature exposures from 68°F (20°C) down to freezing. To prevent this problem, avoid nonbreathing (rubber) footwear when possible, dry the feet and change wool or polypro socks when feet become wet or sweaty (every three to four hours, if necessary), and periodically elevate, air, dry, and massage the feet to promote circulation. Avoid tight, constrictive clothing. At night footwear must absolutely be removed and socks changed to dry ones, or simply remove socks and dry the feet before retiring to the sleeping bag.

There are two clinical stages of immersion foot. In the initial stage the foot is cold, swollen, waxy, and mottled with dark burgundy to blue splotches. This foot is spongy to touch, whereas the frozen foot is very hard. Skin is sodden and friable. Loss of feeling makes walking difficult. The second stage lasts from days to weeks. The feet are swollen, red, and hot. Blisters form and infection and gangrene are common problems. The pain from immersion foot can be lifelong and massive tissue injury can easily develop.

Treatment: Provide the victim with 650 mg of aspirin every six hours to promote blood circulation. This injury is the only wilderness situation in which drinking alcohol plays a proper role. Provide 1½ ounces of hard liquor every hour while awake and 2 ounces every two hours during sleeping hours; this helps dilate the blood vessels and increase the flow of blood to the feet. Immediate stretcher evacuation is necessary.

Other cold injuries, such as chilblains, are less threatening and will not seriously injure trip participants. A full discussion of the prevention, diagnosis, and treatment of cold injuries is beyond the scope of this book, but you can find full details in my book *Basic Essentials Hypothermia (see appendix B)*.

HEAT CRAMPS

Salt depletion can result in nausea, twitching of muscle groups, and at times severe cramping of abdominal muscles, legs, or elsewhere. Treatment consists of stretching the muscles involved (avoid overly aggressive massage), resting in a cool environment, and replacing salt losses. Generally ⅓ to ½ ounce (10 to 15 grams) of salt and generous water replacement should be adequate treatment.

HEAT EXHAUSTION

Heat exhaustion is a classic example of shock, but in this case one encountered while working in a hot environment and due to a heat stress injury. The body has dilated the blood vessels in the skin, attempting to divert heat from the core to the surface for cooling. However, this dilation is so pronounced, coupled with profuse sweating and loss of fluid—also a part of the cooling process—that the blood pressure to the entire system falls too low to adequately supply the brain and other organs. The patient will have a rapid heart rate and will have the other symptoms associated with shock: pale color, nausea, dizziness, headache, and a light-headed feeling. Generally the patient is sweating profusely, but this may not be the case. Skin temperature may be low, normal, or only mildly elevated.

Treatment: Treat for shock. Have the patient lie down immediately, elevate the feet to increase the blood supply to the head, and cover if body temperature is cool or the skin clammy. Also provide copious water; ⅓ to ½ ounce (10 to 15 grams) of salt would also be helpful, but water is the most important. Give a minimum of 1 to 2 quarts (0.9 to 1.8 liters). Obviously, fluids can only be administered if the patient is conscious. If unconscious, elevate the feet 3 feet (0.9 meters) above head level and try to protect from the potential of accidentally inhaling vomit.

HEAT STROKE

Heat stroke, or sunstroke as it is also called, represents the complete breakdown of the heat-control process (thermal regulation). There is a total loss of the ability to sweat. Core temperatures rise over 105°F (40.5°C) and will soon exceed 115°F (46°C) and result in death if this condition is not treated aggressively. THIS IS A TRUE MEDICAL EMERGENCY. The patient will be confused and rapidly become unconscious.

Treatment: Immediately move the victim into shade or erect a hasty barrier for shade. Cool by spraying the victim with water and fanning. Massage limbs to allow the cooler blood of the extremities to return to core circulation more readily. Sacrifice your water supply, if necessary even urinate on the victim, fan and massage to provide the best coolant effect possible. **Evacuate:** This person's temperature regulation will be quite unstable for an unknown length of time. She is critically ill and needs to be hospitalized as soon as possible.

PRICKLY HEAT

This is a heat rash caused by the entrapment of sweat in glands in the skin. This can result in irritation and frequently severe itching.

Treatment: Cool and dry the involved area, avoiding conditions that may induce sweating for a while. Topical medications are less effective than the steps just mentioned, but from the medical kit apply 1 percent hydrocortisone cream every six hours.

SUNBURN

Prevention of sunburn is particularly important in children, as sun damage sustained before the age of eighteen puts the person at a high risk for the development of malignant melanoma skin cancer in later years. Sun damage is a concern for any age group, as basal cell cancer, squamous cell cancer, and aging of the skin are all associated with burning.

The mainstay of skin protection is through the use of adequate SPF factors in sunblock. But all sunblock is not created equal. New technology in sunblock base is the most important consideration. Most waterproof sunblocks are wax-based formulas. These normally contain one or more forms of parabeen. They clog pores and increase the chance of hyperthermia, and they leave a filmy residue on equipment. It is best to use the new bonding base formulas, such as the Sawyer brand sunblock. This product adheres to the dead epidermis, or outer layer of skin. This allows the skin to breathe, is highly abrasion resistant, and does not come off onto equipment.

Treatment: Manage sunburn as a first-degree burn, with cooling, Spenco 2nd Skin (if you have enough), and moisturizing cream. Aloe vera is an excellent anti-inflammation agent to use.

CHAPTER EIGHTEEN

Lightning

A single lightning strike often injures or kills more than one person. It kills or injures from a direct strike, from ground current, from splash current ricocheting off a nearby object such as a fence, or from the blast of exploding air. Amazingly only about one-third of lightning victims are killed, but two-thirds of the survivors suffer significant injuries. While multiple organ systems may be injured, the lightning may not actually penetrate but may rather "flash over" the patient's skin, since current travels over the surface of a conductor.

Figure 21
A cone of protection exists around a tall object. This position is in the area under a 45-degree angle drawn from the top of the object to the ground. Position yourself within the cone, but not too near the outer edge or too close to the object. Lightning can jump from a tree, a cliff face, or other object to you.

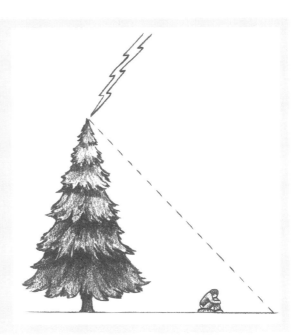

To diminish the chance of getting struck, try to stay in the "cone of protection" (see figure 21). Squat on the ground on an insulated pad. Keep your feet together to lessen the chance of ground current shock. Hold your mouth open to diminish air pressure damage to your eardrums in case of a close strike. Spread out a group but stay close enough to maintain visual or verbal contact with each other. If boating, attempt to get to shore, waves and shoreline permitting. Otherwise maneuver to prevent swamping and keep as low in the boat as possible to decrease the boat's center of gravity and to decrease the chance of attracting a direct lightning strike.

Treatment: Provide CPR (see page 12). Protect the neck and back from possible fractures (see page 40). **Evacuate** all patients surviving a lightning strike for definitive medical evaluation and treatment.

CHAPTER NINETEEN

Insects

Insects are capable of providing us with our most memorable outdoor moments. In fact they are capable of taking the "great" out of the great outdoors. They are also capable of making us ill and giving us allergic reactions that range from local discomfort to life threatening. One of the most important outdoor skills is learning how to keep insects off of us. Modern technology has provided us with some wonderful techniques.

Treat your clothing with a spray of 0.5 percent permethrin, which is available at most outdoor sporting goods stores. This is one of the most important precautions that you can take toward staying well in the outdoors. The proper technique is to spray your camp clothes, even your tent netting, with enough permethrin to lightly dampen the material. Let dry overnight. This substance will not be absorbed through your skin, and it is very rare to have sensitivity to it. It will not harm fabrics. It will kill ticks and chiggers before they have a chance to attach to you for about a two-week period—long enough to consider changing your clothes anyway. It will also decrease the number of insects that will land on your clothing, although it will not totally prevent bites from flying insects.

To prevent insect bites you should apply a DEET lotion to your skin. A new technology—encapsulated DEET—has been developed to provide efficient and safe delivery of DEET. There is minimal skin absorption with this new repellent, available from Sawyer Products in a long-lasting 20 percent formulation.

Deet is a fairly poor blackfly repellent. This is one reason that high concentrations of DEET became popular several years ago. Fairly large amounts of DEET are absorbed through the skin; in fact about 17 percent of the DEET that you apply to your skin surface (of a high-concentration preparation) comes out in your urine. Skin absorbs less of lower concentrations of DEET, unless you have to apply them repeatedly. A composite formulation, containing low amounts of DEET and a blackfly repellent, solve the problem of providing fly and mosquito protection with very little absorption by the skin.

There is a role for 100 percent DEET and that is in the treatment of head or body netting. The best body netting is a loose weave that really isn't netting at all, but a cloth garment that allows air to flow freely (a great advantage on hot summer days). The cloth absorbs the DEET and provides about two days of significant protection before retreatment. The best method of applying this material is to seal the garment in a polyethylene zip-top bag, pour in about an ounce of 100 percent DEET, and leave overnight.

Treatment: The pain of stings and local skin reactions to bites can be helped with almost any pain reliever or anti-itch medicine applied locally. The best choices are cold packs or damp towels that will cool as they evaporate; 1 percent hydrocortisone cream from the medical kit; or cold tea bags from the kitchen kit. A thin paste of baking powder also works, as does Adolph's Meat Tenderizer. Oral antihistamine, such as Benadryl, helps with the reaction. Oral pain medication will help with both pain and itch.

ANAPHYLACTIC SHOCK/ALLERGIC REACTIONS

While most commonly due to insect stings, anaphylactic shock may result from a serious allergic reaction to medications, shellfish, and other foods—in fact to anything. We are not born sensitive to these things but become allergic with repeated exposures. Those developing anaphylaxis are generally warned of their severe sensitivity by welts (urticaria) that form all over their body immediately after exposure, the development of an asthmatic attack with respiratory wheezing, or the onset of symptoms of shock.

Treatment: While these symptoms normally develop within two hours, and certainly before twelve hours, this deadly form of shock can begin within seconds of exposure. It cannot be treated as indicated in the section on "normal" shock on page 7. The antidote for anaphylactic shock is a prescription drug called epinephrine (Adrenaline). It is available for emergency use in a special automatic syringe called the EpiPen (figure 22). The normal dose is 0.3 cc for an adult of the 1:1000 epinephrine solution given "subQ" (in the fatty layer beneath the skin). While it is not necessary to treat the itchy, generalized rash, the epinephrine should be given if the voice becomes husky (signifying swelling of the airway) and if wheezing or shock occurs. This injection may

Figure 22
The EpiPen is used to treat severe allergic reactions.

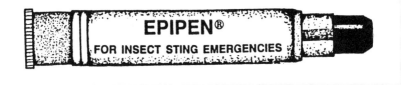

EPIPEN®
FOR INSECT STING EMERGENCIES

have to be repeated in fifteen to twenty minutes if the symptoms return. Antihistamines are of no value in treating the shock or asthmatic component of anaphylaxis, but antihistamines can help prevent delayed allergic swelling and may protect against irregular heartbeats.

The epinephrine dose for persons under twelve years of age is one-half the adult dose, which can be given by using the automatic injection EpiPen Jr .

Evacuate anyone experiencing anaphylactic reactions even though he has responded to the epinephrine. He is at risk of the condition returning, and he must be monitored carefully over the next twenty-four hours. People can die of anaphylaxis very quickly, even in spite of aggressive medical support in a hospital emergency department. After twenty-four hours he is no longer at risk of an anaphylactic reaction, and if there are no symptoms, the evacuation can be terminated.

NO-SEE-UMS AND BITING GNATS

These two examples of insect life are the scourge of the north country, or any country in which they may be found. Many local people refer to any small blackfly as a "no-see-um," but the true bugs by that name are, indeed, very hard to see. They usually come out on a hot, sticky night. The attack is sudden and feels like fire over your entire exposed body surface area. Under the careful examination of a flashlight, you will notice incredibly small gnats struggling with their heads down, biting fiercely. This is the perfect time to apply some of the protein-encapsulated DEET. Lacking that, any DEET solution will do. One thing that doesn't work much of the time is mosquito netting as these small creatures can fly right through it. Immersion in cold water will help relieve symptoms temporarily, at least until your skin warms up above freezing and then you can feel the fire again.

Gnats, on the other hand, are a small blackfly whose bite is seldom felt. But these gentle biters leave behind a red, pimplelike lesion to remind you of their visit. A rash of these pimples around the neck and ankles attests to their ability to sneak through protective clothing.

Treatment: Severe cases require Benadryl 25 mg every six hours. An application of 1 percent dibucaine ointment provides local relief. If your medical kit lacks these items, make a cold poultice from wet tea bags and apply to the wounds. This draws the inflammation to a head and soothes the wounds.

BLACKFLIES

DEET compounds will prevent bites, but the concentration must be 30 percent or greater and even the pure formula will work only a short time. It is best to use a specific blackfly repellent or a composite formula of blackfly repellent with low amounts of DEET. For years Skin-So-Soft bath oil, marketed by Avon, has been mentioned as a blackfly repellent. It does work, but it requires frequent applications, approximately every fifteen minutes. Netting and heavy clothes that can be sealed at the cuffs may be required. All blackfly species like to land and crawl, worming their way under and through protective clothing and netting. Spray clothing and netting with 0.5 percent permethrin as mentioned in the next section on mosquitoes.

Treatment: Blackfly bites can result in nasty sores that are usually self-limited although at times slow healing. If infection is obvious, treat as indicated in the section on puncture wounds on page 20. Dibucaine ointment 1 percent will provide local pain relief. Benadryl 25 mg every six hours reduces swelling and itch.

MOSQUITOES

Adequate mosquito netting for the head and for the tent or cot while sleeping is essential. Spraying netting and clothing with 0.5 percent permethrin increases the effectiveness of the netting and decreases bug bites enormously. Permethrin is an insecticide, not a repellent. It kills mosquitoes, ticks, blackflies, and other biting insects but *does not* chase them away. Do not apply to skin. It is not harmful to your skin, but the skin deactivates this substance and prevents it from working.

I have not found Vitamin B1 (thiamin) to be an effective oral agent for preventing mosquito bites. Nor have I found that electronic sound devices to repel these critters have ever dented mosquito buzzing or biting enthusiasm.

Treatment: A considerable number of bites, or sensitivity to bites, may require an antihistamine, such as Benadryl 25 mg, and Dibucaine ointment 1 percent; both used every six hours can provide local itch relief.

TICKS

More vector-borne diseases are transmitted in the United States by ticks than by any other agent. Ticks must have blood meals to survive their various transformations. It is during these meals that disease can be transmitted to humans and other animals. Two families of ticks can transmit disease to humans: the Ixodidae, or hard ticks, and the Argasidae, or soft ticks. The life cycle of the hard ticks takes two years to complete, including the egg, the six-legged larva or seed tick, the eight-legged immature nymph, and the eight-legged mature adult. They must remain attached for hours to days while obtaining their blood meal. Disease will not be transferred if the tick can be removed before forty-eight hours. The soft ticks can live many years without food. They have several nymph stages and may take multiple blood meals. They usually stay attached less than thirty minutes. Of the soft ticks, only the genus *Ornithodoros* transmit disease in the United States, namely relapsing fever. The forty-eight-hour rule does not apply in this case.

Prevention of attachment is the best defense against tick-borne disease. DEET insect repellents are very effective against ticks. Permethrin 0.5 percent spray on clothing kills ticks upon contact. The combination of permethrin on clothing and DEET on skin is 100 percent effective against tick attachment.

Treatment: How do you remove a tick? A tried-and-true method is to grasp the skin around the insertion of the tick with a pair of fine-point tweezers and pull straight outward, removing the tick and a chunk of skin. For some reason this doesn't hurt. Four commercial tick-removing devices that do a decent job removing ticks are sold under the brand names of the Tick Nipper, the Tick Plier, the Original Ticked Off, and the Pro-Tick Remedy. Hot wires, matches, glue, fingernail polish, Vaseline—all do not work. Burning the tick might cause it to vomit germs right into the victim, yet it will not let go. Be careful not to grasp the tick body. Crushing it might also cause germs to be injected into the victim. Contact a physician after your return home for further treatment advice.

CATERPILLAR AND MILLIPEDE REACTIONS

The puss caterpillar (*Megalopyge opercularis*) of the southern United States and the gypsy moth caterpillar (*Lymantria dispar*) of the northeastern states have bristles that cause an almost immediate skin rash and welt formation.

Treatment includes patting the victim with a piece of adhesive tape to remove these bristles. Taking Benadryl and coating the area with 1 percent hydrocortisone cream relieves the irritation. Millipedes do not bite, but contact can cause skin irritation. Cold packs can reduce discomfort. Wash thoroughly.

CENTIPEDE BITES

Some of the larger centipedes can inflict a painful bite that causes a local swelling and painful, red lesion. Treatment with a cold pack is usually sufficient. Some bites are severe and cause swelling of the lymph nodes at the joints along the blood-flow pattern toward the heart from the bite site. Swelling at the bite location may persist for weeks.

Treatment: Use pain medication and apply dibucaine ointment.

ANT OR FIRE ANT

While many ants can alert you to their presence with a burning bite, fire ants can produce an intensely painful bite that pales to insignificance due to a surrounding cluster of stings. While holding on tightly with his biting pincer and pivoting around, the ant then stings repeatedly in as many places as the stinger can reach, causing a cluster of small, painful blisters to appear. These can take eight to ten days to heal.

Treatment: Use cold packs, damp cloth for evaporative cooling, and pain medication. Large local reactions may require an antihistamine such as Benadryl 25 mg, two capsules every six hours, and even prescription steroid medication. Local application of dibucaine ointment 1 percent can provide some relief. The greatest danger is to the hypersensitive individual who may have an anaphylactic reaction. This should be treated as indicated under anaphylactic shock, page 66.

SCORPION STING

Most North American scorpion stings are relatively harmless. Stings usually cause only localized pain and slight swelling. The wound may feel numb.

Treatment: Benadryl and Percogesic may be all that is required for treatment. A cold pack will help relieve local pain.

The potentially lethal *Centruroides sculptuatus* is the exception to this rule. This yellow-colored scorpion lives in Mexico, New Mexico, Arizona, and the California side of the Colorado River. The sting causes immediate, severe pain with swelling and subsequent numbness. The neurotoxin injected with this bite may cause respiratory failure. Respiratory assistance may be required (see page 12). Tapping on the wound lightly with your finger will cause the patient to withdraw due to severe pain. This is an unusual reaction and does not occur with most insect stings.

   Treatment: A specific antivenin is available in Mexico and is also produced by the Poisonous Animals Laboratory at Arizona State University for local use. In addition to the antivenin, other prescription medications may be required to help control the pain and spasm.

SPIDER BITES

Generally spiders will make a solitary bite rather than several. If a person awakens with multiple bites, he has probably collided with some other arthropod. While only some spiders are considered poisonous, all spiders have venom that will cause local tissue inflammation and even slight necrosis or destruction. Most spiders are unable to bite well enough to inject the venom.

BLACK WIDOW

The black widow *(Latrodectus mactans)* is generally glossy black with a red hourglass mark on the abdomen. Sometimes the hourglass mark is merely a red dot or the two parts of the hourglass do not connect. At times the coat is not shiny and it may contain white. The bite may only be a pinprick, but generally a dull cramping pain begins within one quarter of an hour, and this may spread gradually until it involves the entire body. The muscles may go into spasms and the abdomen becomes boardlike. Extreme restlessness is typical. The pain can be excruciating. Nausea, vomiting, swelling of eyelids, weakness, anxiety, and painful breathing may all develop. A healthy adult can usually survive, with the pain abating in several hours and the remaining symptoms disappearing in several days.

   Treatment: An ice cube on the bite, if available, may reduce local pain. A specific antidote is available at an emergency room of a hospital, where other prescription medications can also be given to reduce the muscle spasm and pain. Percogesic or ibuprofen may be used to treat the pain.

BROWN RECLUSE

A brown coat with a black violin marking on the top of the body identifies this spider *(Loxosceles reclusa)*. The initial bite is mild and may be overlooked at the time. In an hour or two, a slight redness may appear; by several hours a small bleb appears at the bite site. At times the wound begins to appear as a bull's eye with several rings of red and blanched circles around the bite. The bleb ruptures, forming a crust, which then sloughs off; then a large necrotic ulcer forms that gradually enlarges. Over the first thirty-six hours, vomiting, fever, skin rash, and joint pain may develop, and a decrease in the ability of blood to clot can result in bleeding and bruising.

Treatment: Apply ice to the wound as soon as possible. An antivenin has been developed, and other prescription medications are available. Prophylactic use of antibiotics has been recommended. Avoid the application of heat to this wound, even though it is inflamed and necrotic. Give four tablets of ibuprofen 200 mg every six hours to help with pain and to reduce inflammation. Apply triple-antibiotic ointment and cover with Spenco 2nd Skin dressing.

CHAPTER TWENTY

Snakebites

Prevention is easier than treatment. Wear boots that cover the ankle and avoid reaching into areas where your view is obstructed in habitats of poisonous snakes. Avoid snakes when seen rather than try to kill them. These steps will prevent most snakebite incidents from happening.

NONPOISONOUS SNAKEBITE

Get away from the snake. Cleanse the bitten area with surgical cleaner or soap and water. Treat for shock. Manage the wound as a puncture wound (see page 20).

POISONOUS SNAKEBITE

Not everyone bitten by a poisonous snake will have venom injected. Fully 20 percent of rattlesnake and 30 percent of cottonmouth water moccasin and copperhead snakebites do not have evidence of any venom. If the snake injects venom, the first symptom noted by many is a peculiar tingling in the mouth, often associated with a rubbery or metallic taste. This symptom may develop in minutes and long before any swelling occurs at the bite site. Envenomation may produce instant burning pain. Weakness, sweating, nausea, and fainting may occur either with poisonous or nonpoisonous snakebites, simply due to the trauma of being bitten. In case of envenomation, within one hour there will generally be swelling, pain, tingling, and/or numbness at the bite site. As several hours pass, bruising and discoloration of the skin begins and becomes progressively worse. Blisters may form that are sometimes filled with blood. Chills and fever may begin, followed by muscle tremor, decrease in blood pressure, headache, blurred vision, and bulging eyes. The surface blood vessels may fill with blood clots, and this can lead to significant tissue damage after several days.

Treatment: Immobilize the injured part at heart level or slightly below. Do not make a cut at the bite site. Do not apply cold—this is associated with increased tissue damage. Treat for shock (see page 7) and **evacuate** to professional medical help.

Evacuate: There is a golden hour and a half before the effects of North American pit viper venom causes significant effects that might make the victim nonambulatory. You might want to start walking the victim towards the road head to shorten the length of a possible litter evacuation in case the victim does get quite ill. This walkout should be performed in a calm, but urgent manner. If the patient is small and lightweight, you can carry her out. Attempting to carry a heavy victim would slow down the evacuation, whereas her walking out will not significantly increase the spread of venom. Some people mistakenly believe you should carry the person out so that she will have a lower pulse rate and thus the blood will not move the venom around so quickly. The point I always make is that the person who has been bitten has a rapid pulse rate—even when lying perfectly still—because she is scared. The venom is slowly diffusing away from the bite site anyway. In contrast, the calming effect of someone having applied the above first-aid procedures and then walking toward home and professional care will probably reduce the heart rate along with the anxiety for both victim and rescuers.

Patient Name _____ Age _____ Sex _____

Date/Time of Accident _____

Weather: Temp _____ Rain/Snow _____ Visibility _____ Wind _____ (mph)

Type of illness or injury: _____

Is patient on medication/drugs? _____

Physical examination findings: _____

_____

_____

Can patient eat, drink? _____ Last food intake _____ Allergies _____

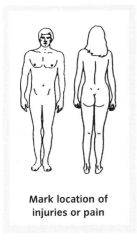

Mark location of injuries or pain

Primary Survey: Survey the scene for additional hazards; check the airway; check circulation; protect the neck.

Secondary Survey: *Head*—look for wounds, fluid coming from eyes, nose, ears, mouth; check level of consciousness (alert, only responds to verbal, only responds to pain, or unresponsive).

Neck—is airway OK; pain along spine to touch

Chest—compress ribs from side, any pain or deformity

Abdomen—press gently, any spasm, distension, pain

Back—touch along the spine, note point tenderness

Pelvis—cup crest of hip and press gently downward toward midline of body looking for instability or pain

Legs—squeeze each one from groin to toes looking for lack of circulation, sensation, or motion in toes

We require (tents, clothing, medical supplies, food) _____

_____

_____

Our location is: _____

Our plan is to: _____

On the reverse indicate medical experience/training/number of party members who can help, days of food on hand. Draw a map of location or intended route.

Appendix B
For More Information

BOOKS

Forgey, William W., *Basic Essentials Hypothermia*, second edition (Guilford, Conn.: Globe Pequot, 1999).

_____, *Wilderness Medical Society Practice Guidelines for Wilderness Emergency Care*, fifth edition (Guilford, Conn.: Globe Pequot, 2006).

_____, *Wilderness Medicine*, fifth edition (Guilford, Conn.: Globe Pequot, 1999).

Tilton, Buck, *Wilderness First Responder*, second edition (Guilford, Conn.: Globe Pequot, 2004).
_____, and Frank Hubbell. *Medicine for the Backcountry,* third edition (Guilford, Conn.: Globe Pequot, 1999).

WEB SITES

William Forgey, MD: www.docforgey.com or www.docforgeytravelmedicine.com

Wilderness Medical Society: www.wms.org

About the Author

William Forgey is engaged in the full-time practice of family medicine in Merrill-ville, Indiana. He is a member of the board of trustees of the International Association for Medical Assistance to Travelers (IAMAT), a fellow of the Explorer's Club, a lecturer on medical care in high-risk recreation at several universities, and a leader of summer and winter expeditions into northern Canada. A former Boy Scout scoutmaster and Medical Explorer Post and High Adventure Explorer Post advisor, Dr. Forgey currently serves on the National Health and Safety Committee and as an advisory board member for the Northern Tier High Adventure Base for the Boy Scouts of America. He is the national consultant for the Student Conservation Association and many other nonprofit organizations. He was named as one of America's twenty greatest living explorers by the Explorers Club in New York City and, as such, had a subcamp named for him at the National Boy Scout Jamboree in 2005.

He is the author of fourteen wilderness medicine and camping books and a contributor to the current edition of the *Field Book,* published by the Boy Scouts of America; to *The Wilderness Educator,* a textbook for outdoor educators; and to several other books.